Nursing Care Planning Guides
Set 1
Second Edition

Margo Creighton Neal, RN, MN
VICE PRESIDENT, WILLIAMS & WILKINS

Patricia Feltz Cohen, RN, MA, EdM
CONSULTANT, HUNTINGTON BEACH, CA

Phyllis Gorney Cooper, RN, MN
CONSULTANT, LOS ANGELES, CA

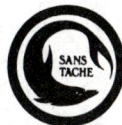

SANS TACHE

WILLIAMS & WILKINS
Baltimore • London • Los Angeles • Sydney

Copyright © 1980—Margo Creighton Neal
Copyright © 1985—Williams & Wilkins
428 East Preston Street, Baltimore, Maryland 21202 U.S.A.

Printed in the United States of America

Library of Congress Cataloging in Publication Data

Main entry under title:
Nursing care planning guides, set 1, 2nd Ed.

    1. Nursing—Handbooks, manuals, etc. 2. Nursing—Planning—Handbooks, manuals, etc. I. Neal, Margo Creighton, 1935–   , joint author. II. Cohen, Patricia Feltz, 1932–   , joint author. III. Cooper, Phyllis Gorney, 1946–   , joint author. IV. Title.
RT51.N36   1980   610.73   80-16417
ISBN 0-683-09519-6

   86 87 88 89   10 9 8 7 6 5

PREFACE

This second edition of Nursing Care Planning Guides, Set 1, has been revised to help you write complete and useful nursing care plans.

With increasing emphasis on written care plans as a tool for accountability and evidence of planning, these Guides can also help nurses establish criteria for nursing audit.

This revised edition contains all goals and objectives in terms of patient behaviors or expected outcomes of care. The categories of patient problems have been revised to reflect the growing use of nursing diagnoses, and the references lists have been updated.

In this edition, we attempted to avoid stereotyping the nurse as "she" and the patient as "he" by using "s/he" in lieu of she/he. However, the English language has not yet produced a combination form for masculine and feminine pronouns, thus you will note some referral to the patient in the masculine form only.

Margo C. Neal
Patricia F. Cohen
Phyllis G. Cooper

FOREWORD

Each of these Nursing Care Planning Guides is written in the format of a nursing care plan and contains all the basic components: long-term goals, areas of patient problems, patient outcomes, and nursing actions.

It is expected that the nurse will assess the "specific considerations" category (e.g. fluids and electrolytes) and if there is a problem, define it specifically (e.g. dehydration); then select a patient outcome and nursing actions from those suggested on the Guide. Not all of the suggested outcomes and actions will be appropriate for each patient.

Additional information is also provided for the nurses' own use: definition and general considerations of the condition, nursing responsibilities, and recommended references.

To use these Guides most efficiently, scan the Table of Contents. Note that this Set is comprised of three sections: A) med-surg conditions; B) patient behaviors; and C) supplementary information. You may wish to consult more than one Guide per patient. For example, a patient is depressed following an ileostomy. Read, "The Patient with an Ileostomy (#1:13), "The Patient Experiencing Depression" (#1:26), and "Basic Principles for Changing A Temporary or Permanent Appliance (#1:43).

This Set is also cross-referenced to three additional Sets of Nursing Care Planning Guides, Sets 2, 3, and 4. For detailed information on each condition, consult med-surg texts.

Nursing Care Planning Guides should be used as guidelines and ready-references only, not as standard care plans. To use them as the latter negates individual differences in patients, thus contradicting the original purpose of care plans . . . i.e. individualized patient care.

Set No. 1
TABLE OF CONTENTS

A—Medical & Surgical Conditions

1. Patient with a CVA (Cerebral Vascular Accident): Early Acute Phase
2. Patient with a CVA (Cerebral Vascular Accident): Convalescent Phase
3. Patient with Cholecystectomy
4. Patient with Cirrhosis of the Liver
5. Patient with a Colostomy
6. Patient with Congestive Heart Failure: Chronic Phase
7. Patient with Diabetes
8. Patient with Emphysema: Pulmonary
9. Patient with Hemorrhoidectomy
10. Patient with Hepatitis
11. Patient with Hypertension
12. Patient with a Hysterectomy
13. Patient with an Ileostomy
14. Patient with a Mastectomy
15. Patient with a Peptic Ulcer: Medical Management
16. Patient with a Peptic Ulcer: Surgical Management
17. Patient with Pneumonia
18. Patient with Rheumatoid Arthritis
19. Patient with a Thoracotomy

B—Patient Behaviors

20. The Patient Manifesting Aggression
21. The Patient Manifesting Anger
22. The Patient Experiencing Anxiety
23. The Patient Experiencing Confusion
24. The Patient Manifesting Denial
25. The Patient Experiencing Dependency
26. The Patient Experiencing Depression
27. Dealing with Impending Death
28. The Patient Experiencing Fear
29. The Patient Displaying Manipulation
30. The Patient Experiencing Pain
31. Responses to Loss: The Grief and Mourning Process
32. The Patient Experiencing Sensory Disturbances
33. The Patient in Shock, Psychogenic

C—Supplementary Information

34. Chest Tubes and Bottles: Water-Seal Drainage
35. Diabetes: Differentiating Hypoglycemia and Ketoacedosis
36. Diabetes: General Dietary Principles
37. Diabetes: Liquid Diet Substitutes
38. Diabetes: Properties of Insulin Preparations
39. Diabetes: Recommended Care of the Feet
40. Effects of Hospitalization: Part A: Tension-Producing Causes
41. Effects of Hospitalization: Part B: Assessment
42. Effects of Hospitalization: Part C: Prolonged Confinement
43. Basic Principles for Changing an . . . Appliance
44. Interviewing: Suggestions for
45. Mastectomy: Arm Exercises
46. Nursing Assessment Form: "RESTORING +"
47. Range of Motion Exercises
48. Steps in Writing Nursing Care Plans
49. Teaching Patients: General Suggestions
50. Teaching Patients: Specific Plan for Skills and Procedures

The Patient with a CVA (Cerebral-Vascular Accident):
Early, Acute Phase

Definition: A cerebral vascular accident or stroke is an interruption in the intracerebral circulation related to a condition of vascular insufficiency, a thrombosis, an embolism, or a hemorrhage.

LONG TERM GOAL: The patient will have the cause and extent of damage determined; the patient will wish to recover and will accept a comprehensive, active rehabilitation program aimed at independent functioning.

General Considerations:

— **Incidence:** Stroke is the third leading cause of death in the U.S. Although mortality rate of patients during acute phase (24 hrs. to 2 wks.) is very high, those who survive this crisis should not be regarded as hopeless or permanently helpless. Even the most severely paralyzed patients, or the most neglected and deformed patients can be taught some means of self-help and self-esteem.

— **Signs & Symptoms:** Headache, vomiting, fever, nuchal (neck) rigidity, hypertension, mental changes, confusion, coma, hemiplegia, and speech disturbances.

— **Diagnostic Work-up** entails a general physical and history, a complete neurological exam, and laboratory and x-ray studies.

— **Treatment is aimed** at prevention of complications, during acute phase, which result in severe disability or death, and, after the acute phase, comprehensive rehabilitation to regain independent functioning with minimum possible residual deficits.

— **Successful rehabilitation** is one that is adequately planned and implemented as soon as possible. It involves the active participation and enthusiastic cooperation of the patient, his family, his physician, the nursing staff, and other medical specialists in the health agency and community. It requires a team approach and an attitude of optimism tempered with realism, gentle empathy yet firmness, technical skill and knowledge with compassion.

Specific Considerations, Potential Patient Outcomes, and Nursing Actions:

1) Mental Status and Cardio-vascular Function   The patient's current status and problems are assessed; the patient maintains appropriate level of consciousness and adequate circulation:

— interview, examine, observe & assess whether pt. is alert, lethargic, somnolent, stuporous or comatose, oriented or disoriented, judgment sound or impaired; note responses to orientation questions & simple commands;

— note & record magnitude, duration & time when any changes in the above status occur;

— take & record vital signs at least every hour to note developing complications as soon as possible; note pupillary reaction to light, BP in both arms, apical & radial pulse rate, quality & rhythm of respiration, body temperature;

— avoid oversedation & help keep pt. oriented to time & surroundings;

— note & report changes in pt.'s blood gases & electrolyte studies;
— examine & report signs of peripheral stasis in extremities (cyanosis, edema, coldness); determine area & degree of paralysis & sensory loss.

2) Respiratory Function

The patient maintains a patent airway and pulmonary ventilation is improved; the patient removes or is assisted to remove accumulated bronchial secretions; the patient is free of hypoxia and pneumonia:
— place pt. in a side-lying position on a level bed, with head slightly extended & turned to side to lessen danger of aspiration;
— turn hourly; perform deep breathing exercises & assist pt. to cough up loosened secretions;
— aspirate secretions with nasopharyngeal suctioning if above measures are ineffective;
— consider need for IPPB, oxygen therapy and/or ventilation assistance; discuss with physician & arrange PRN;
— keep paralyzed tongue from obstructing pharynx with plastic airway;
— observe for signs of hypoxia (restlessness, cyanosis, respiratory distress, increased pulse rate);
— discuss with physician need for medication to liquefy secretions & give as ordered.

3) Positioning and Safety

The patient is protected from injuries and compromised cardiopulmonary function; the patient is free of preventable complications of immobility (e.g. edema, contractures, deformities, subluxation of affected shoulder, pneumonia, thrombophlebitis and skin breakdown); the patient's musculoskeletal system is maintained functionally:
— maintain therapeutic body alignment with head, shoulders & hips level on a firm mattress with bed board;
— brace feet against footboard, in line with legs, heels off mattress & protected from pressure;
— use trochanter roll to maintain neutral position of hip (neither external nor internal rotation), and to help prevent pain & discomfort;
— support arms & hands in functional positions: slightly flexed at elbow, extended wrists & a *hard* hand roll or rubber ball to keep fingers in "grasp" position & to control spasm; elevate affected hand to prevent dependent edema; (sometimes plaster or plastic hand & wrist splints are used to lessen contracture development);
— change position at least Q2H; use prone or Sim's position but limit time spent on affected side;
— use padded side rails & protective vest restraints if needed; keep a tongue blade or airway at bedside for possible seizures.

4) Activity (Rest and Exercise)

The patient will maintain adequate cerebral blood flow, protected from increased intravascular pressure and further damage to body system:
— maintain complete bed rest for at least 48 hrs. or until condition & vital signs stabilize;
— avoid unnecessary transportation of patient for tests which can be done at bedside; assist technicians so that pt. is disturbed minimally;

— provide all physical care, so that pt. can really rest; try to reduce restlessness by having a family member or friend present; encourage stroking, touching or hand holding to provide reassuring comfort & physical as well as emotional relaxation; administer sedatives & tranquilizers PRN;

— if stroke was NOT due to hemorrhage, perform **full range of motion exercises passively to both sides,** affected & unaffected, from the outset; otherwise these are begun when doctor feels that danger of re-bleeding is past; refer to NCPG #1:47, "Range of Motion Exercises";

— as soon as possible, begin teaching pt. how to move in bed with use of trapeze & foot-of-bed pull rope; when condition permits, teach pt. & family transfer techniques, stressing safety factors; consult with physical therapist; evaluate tolerance levels; encourage sitting, standing, locomotion or in-bed exercises that are in keeping with pt. progress & activity tolerance (fatiguability level).

5) Nutrition, Fluids and Electrolytes

The patient restores and maintains optimal nutritional status, fluid intake and electrolyte balance; the patient's appetite and ability to feed self are restored:

— monitor rate, flow & accurate administration of prescribed IV fluids; refer to NCPG #2:46, "Intravenous Therapy: General Principles";

— maintain accurate intake & output records;

— administer nasogastric tube feedings of liquid nutrients on a regular schedule when ordered; elevate head of bed; observe for aspiration;

— if hyperalimentation therapy used, refer to NCPG #3:50, "Hyperalimentation";

— test swallowing ability periodically; attempt fluid feedings orally when possible; use of a training cup or a rubber tipped syringe may be desirable, as it is often easier to drink and swallow this way than with a straw; nevertheless, be prepared for possible choking; suction PRN;

— advance to soft foods when tolerated, offering them in ways found to be effective; feeding by a family member is often preferable to a busy staff person; teach those feeding pt. to place fingers against the effected side of neck and cheek in order to support flaccid muscles; this will help prevent choking as food must remain on unaffected side to go down safely; do not feed pt. anything that has pits, bones or tough, fibrous pieces;

— attempt to identify food preferences & dislikes to motivate adequate intake; feed several small meals daily rather than larger meals;

— provide oral hygiene after each feeding; add lubricant to lips to prevent dryness & cracking.

6) Elimination   The patient will maintain an adequate elimination, satisfactorily consistent with protection of skin and prevention of infection; the patient will have restored normal bowel and bladder function:
- when possible, try placing pt. on bedpan at frequent, regular intervals to avoid unnecessary catheterization;
- determine whether pt. is aware of need to void; observe for communication signals; check for distention & signs of discomfort or restlessness; keep call bell in unaffected hand or within reach;
- if necessary to keep continent, apply external catheter for most males & Foley catheters for most females; using rigid aseptic technique to prevent infection, keep catheter patent & appropriately taped to leg, in a closed drainage system; refer to NCPG #2:39, "Catheters: Indwelling Urethral"; also see NCPG #2:03, "The Patient for Bladder Retraining";
- ensure adequate fluid intake; check urine for specific gravity, signs of bladder infection;
- administer stool softeners, bulk-forming laxatives, pureed fiber foods;
- check for impaction & give suppositories or enemas (low, retention) PRN;
- check with family for pt.'s previous bowel habits & try to re-establish defecation pattern in hospital; see NCPG #2:04, "The Patient for Bowel Retraining"; know that involuntary BM after first week post CVA can be a poor prognostic sign;
- provide meticulous perineal hygiene, keeping patient clean, dry & free of irritation or skin breakdown.

7) Skin Care   The patient will maintain skin integrity, tone, turgor and circulation; skin breakdown, injury and infection will be prevented; prolonged pressure to bony prominences will be relieved or avoided; all potential pressure sites are clean, dry, free of surface irritants and ventilated with circulating air:
- keep pt.'s skin clean, dry (but sufficiently lubricated), free of pressure & adequately warm; promote circulation with frequent changes of position, massages, suitable room ventilation & loose, absorbent bed-clothing;
- utilize pressure prevention aids (cushions, devices, pads, etc.) currently available & effective;
- refer to NCPG #4:42, "Decubitus Ulcer Care: Prevention and Treatment."

8) Communication The patient will reestablish some means of communication between self and others; the patient will express verbally in addition to nonverbal communication; the patient will recognize and recall familiar objects:
- learn whether pt. has motor (expressive) or sensory (receptive) aphasia, & to what degree, in order to determine what can be expected of him & how best to communicate with him;
- maintain eye-to-eye contact with pt. when speaking;
- use simple, one word commands with gestures or pictures;
- speak slowly & repeat key words; do not speak loudly unless pt. is hard of hearing;
- give pt. time to respond; avoid finishing sentences for him;
- don't assume s/he understands or said what s/he intended to say by placing too much value on "verbal" "yes" or "no" replies to your questions; validate responses with non-verbal behavior assessment;
- use facial expressions & touch to communicate & to prevent some of the pt.'s feelings of social isolation & withdrawal;

— consult with speech therapist for added help;
— refer to NCPG #4:03, "The Patient with Aphasia/Dysphasia."

9) Sensory Disturbances

The patient will cope and adapt effectively to visual deficits and distortions; the patient will be protected from injury due to diminished or absent sensation; the patient will compensate for sensory disturbances:
— take safety precautions & teach them to family, e.g. check bath water temperature, avoid heating pads & hot water bottles, have sufficient help when transferring or ambulating patient to prevent falls;
— observe & assess for visual deficits: diplopia & hemianopia; teach patient to turn head to scan visual field; place objects, call button, tray food on unaffected side; have visitors approach pt. from the unaffected side; position bed in room so that pt. can see those approaching from doorway;
— for diplopia, cover the affected eye with an eye patch or shield; explain the loss of depth perception when one eye is used; help patient gauge distance;
— maintain cleanliness of eyes & have pt. wear prescription glasses if s/he has them;
— provide stimuli for eyes, ears & sense of touch; use clocks, radio, flowers, greeting cards, television, various objects of different textures.

10) Psychosocial Adjustment

The patient will adapt effectively to an altered body image; the patient will express negative feelings openly, gradually expressing hope and confidence; the patient will cooperatively participate in an intensive rehabilitation program:
— explore with pt. & family fears of dying, of loss of independence, of loss of control of body functions, of crippling and permanent disability, of loss of speech; encourage expression of feelings of anger, depression, frustration, anxiety, helplessness, hopelessness; be willing to listen;
— recognize & accept emotional mood swings & ambivalent feelings as normal & to be expected; know that inappropriate behavior is common;
— maintain an optimistic, cheerful, patient, confident, competent, warm & compassionate attitude around pt. & family; nevertheless, be realistic & avoid false reassurance;
— explain all nursing activities, treatments & tests; obtain the family's understanding, acceptance & assistance in all aspects of pt. care planning, implementation & evaluation;
— encourage visitors to help pt. speak again & socialize with them;

— assess for history of mental illness, depression, pre-morbid personality strengths & weaknesses; consult freely with pt.'s closest friends, employer, clergyman or trusted associate; request assistance from other professionals; refer to NCPG #1:31, "Responses to Loss: the Grief and Mourning Process," and NCPG #2:29, "The Patient Experiencing a Body Image Disturbance";

— recognize pt.'s accomplishments; point out improvements in condition; find ways to assure pt. that s/he is valued and responsible.

11) Planning for Discharge or Transfer to Convalescent Facility

The patient and family will be prepared for discharge or transfer, expressing optimism, confidence and willingness to participate in rehabilitation program:

— prepare written reports summarizing completely pt.'s problems, how much progress has been attained, what has been learned by pt. & family, what goals remain to be achieved, and what is the anticipated plan of care;

— try to have a personal consultation with the one who will be most involved in pt.'s care;

— provide family & nursing home staff with helpful booklets about the care of the stroke pt.;

— consult a social worker, community health nurse or rehabilitation specialist PRN;

— refer to NCPG #1:02, "The Patient with a Cerebral-Vascular Accident (Convalescent Phase)."

Recommended References

Aphasia and the Family, Strike Back At Stroke, Strokes: A Guide for the Family, and *Guidelines for the Nursing Care of Stroke Patients* (Report of the Joint Committee for Stroke Facilities). American Heart Assn., 7320 Greenville Ave., Dallas, TX 75231.

"Catheters: Indwelling Urethral." *NCP Guide* #2:39, 2nd Ed., Nurseco, 1980.

"Comeback from Disaster: Helping the Stroke Patient Learn To Help Himself," by Mary Ann Kavchak-Keyes. *Nursing 79*, January 1979:32–35.

"Decubitus Ulcer Care: Prevention and Treatment." *NCP Guide* #4:42, Nurseco, 1978.

"For Me, There's No Such Thing As 'Another CVA' Anymore," by Mary Grens. *RN*, September 1977:85–90.

"Hyperalimentation." *NCP GUIDE* #3:50, Nurseco, 1977.

"Intravenous Therapy: General Principles." *NCP Guide* #2:46, 2nd Ed., Nurseco, 1980.

Language Problems After A Stroke (A Guide for Communication), The American Rehabilitation Foundation, 1800 Chicago Ave., Minneapolis, MN 55404.

"Range of Motion Exercises." *NCP Guide* #1:47, 2nd Ed., Nurseco, 1980.

"Responses to Loss: the Grief and Mourning Process." *NCP Guide* #1:31, 2nd Ed., Nurseco, 1980.

"Stroke! Nursing Insights from a Stroke-Nurse Victim." by Frances McNeil. *RN*, September 1975:75–81.

"Teaching Patients: General Suggestions." *NCP Guide* #1:49, 2nd Ed., Nurseco, 1980.

"The Patient Experiencing a Body Image Disturbance." *NCP Guide* #2:29, 2nd Ed., Nurseco, 1980.

"The Patient for Bladder Retraining." *NCP Guide* #2:03, 2nd Ed., Nurseco, 1980.

"The Patient for Bowel Retraining." *NCP Guide* #2:04, 2nd Ed., Nurseco, 1980.

"The Patient with Aphasia/Dysphasia." *NCP Guide* #4:03, Nurseco, 1978.

"The Patient with a Cerebral-Vascular Accident (Convalescent Phase)." *NCP Guide* #1:02, 2nd Ed., Nurseco, 1980.

The Patient with a CVA (Cerebral-Vascular Accident):
Convalescent Phase

LONG TERM GOAL: The patient will perform activities of daily living with confidence, self-esteem and a measure of independence; the patient will regain optimal level of functioning within a lifestyle adapted to residual disabilities from a stroke; the patient is motivated and able to perform a schedule of activities appropriate to condition and rehabilitation goals.

General Considerations:
— The **effective rehabilitation plan** must be coordinated, consistent and clearly communicated to all participating members, including the patient and family. The (stroke) team approach can work in all hospitals, even those without a special rehabilitation department.
— **Regular**, at least weekly, **evaluations** must accompany cooperative implementation of rehabilitation activities to keep the plan current, workable and appropriate to the patient's needs, problems, abilities and progress. The nurse-coordinator or rehabilitation team leader is responsible for arranging the meetings of consulting specialists.
— Refer to NCPG #1:01, "The Patient with a CVA: Early, Acute Phase," for additional information about stroke and patient care which will not be repeated here. For patients over 60, it may be desirable to meet special needs for remotivation and resocialization. See NCPGs #3:34, "The Aged Patient: Resocialization"; and #4:35, "The Aged Patient: Remotivation."
— **Nursing responsibilities** include physical & physical & psychosocial care, assessment of patient needs, problems & concerns re: rehabilitation activities, patient/family education and, usually, coordination of rehabilitation team effort on behalf of patient.

Specific Considerations, Potential Patient Outcomes, and Nursing Actions:

1) Complete Physical Assessment

The patient will be assessed for full use of capabilities within limitations; the patient will be helped to plan realistically for goal achievement:
— participate in physical assessment of pt.; refer to NCPGs #4:47, 48, 49 & 50, "Physical Assessment: Parts A, B, C, & D";
— learn of any chronic medical problems, past & present; determine their effect on stroke rehabilitation plan;
— review care of patient during acute, early phase post CVA.

2) Complete Mental Assessment

The patient will be helped to learn what s/he needs to know to assume fullest possible self-care and responsibility for rehabilitation:
— refer to NCPG #4:41, "Assessment of Mental Status";
— know which side of brain was affected by stroke & its meaning in terms of functions lost or disabled; (left side: speech & language center, right side: balance and motor perceptual center);

— identify extent of language impairment (receptive or expressive type); determine ability to read & write, to remember, to understand, to reason, to use judgment, to solve problems;
— determine visual acuity & residual deficits;
— assess level of emotional stability or lability;
— refer to NCPG #4:03, "The Patient with Aphasia/Dysphasia"; begin speech therapy with or without therapist; if unavailable on a regular basis; arrange for family members and friends to observe & participate in speech training.

3) Life Style Assessment

The patient will participate in appropriate occupational and diversional therapy; the patient will be prepared for discharge to assume former roles and responsibilities within limitations and necessary modifications:
— inquire about pt.'s role & position in family, religious beliefs & practices, educational background;
— know pt.'s work history;
— identify pt.'s patterns of leisure/recreation (hobbies, sports, cultural interests, etc.);
— identify personality strengths & weaknesses (gregarious or a loner, resourceful or unimaginative, agreeable or disagreeable, complaining worrier or cheerful optimist, conservative or willing to try new ways);
— assess financial status & its meaning for pt.

4) Specialist Consultation

The rehabilitation plan will be developed, implemented and evaluated by all participating specialists and consultants in collaboration with the patient and family:
— discuss results of assessment & read written reports of consultants;
— set goals, specify a sequence of activities and coordinate responsibilities;
— arrange & conduct meetings to evaluate progress; encourage pt. & family to participate actively with comments, suggestions, observations.

5) Patient/Family Teaching Program

The patient/family/friends will develop needed skills, knowledge and self-confidence, demonstrating as well as verbalizing their understanding:
— refer to NCPG #1:49, "Teaching Patients: General Suggestions," and NCPG #1:50, "Teaching Patients: Specific Plan for Skills and Procedures";
— reinforce teaching provided by other therapists (physical, speech, occupational, dietetic, etc.);
— obtain & utilize current materials available cost-free from the local heart association for yourself, colleagues & family members;
— avoid hurrying the pt.; take time to make possible comprehension & successful practice; remember that disability, confusion, fatigue & slow progress make learning difficult & discouraging.

6) Activities of Daily Living

The patient will perform basic ADL with success, self-confidence and some independence:
— begin with familiar, easily accomplished tasks to motivate and reassure pt. (eating, grooming, bathing, & dressing);

arrange for the necessary assistive devices to enable the pt. to function maximally;
— have pt. practice each newly acquired skill until it becomes a habit;
— encourage pt. to use affected extremity in as many tasks as possible;
— teach family of helpful devices to use at home for safety & convenience: slip-on clothing & shoes, velcro fasteners & zipper pulls, long-handled shoe horns, grab bars, hand rails, raised toilet seats, movable shower heads, kitchen aids, etc.;
— keep written record of learning gains.

7) Discharge Planning — The patient and family will have access to continued care and help, according to need, desires and resources:
— plan with family & friends so they will have a respite from burden of care and worry for pt. in order to take care of their needs, restore their spirit, strength & energy;
— plan for referrals with local community agencies for help if needed & wanted with financial, occupational, household, emotional or continuing health problems;
— investigate possibilities for pt. to join an organized community stroke self-help group to meet resocialization needs.

Discharge Planning and Teaching Objectives/Outcomes

1) (Patient/Family/Significant Other) Says s/he realizes that some neurological and residual deficits resulting from the stroke may linger indefinitely, but that rehabilitation to the fullest extent of functioning is primarily own responsibility.
2) States s/he knows medications to be taken, dosage, administration and side effects to be reported to doctor.
3) Has appointment for continuing follow-up medical care as well as referrals for home health nursing services, social service assistance and/or homemaker services as needs and wishes indicate.
4) Has received literature from local heart association for stroke rehabilitation suggestions; has written list of instructions from hospital re: exercises, activities, speech practice, and use of assistive devices for activities of daily living or locomotion assistance.

Recommended References
"Assessment of Mental Status." *NCP Guide #4:41*, Nurseco, 1978.
Do It Yourself Again, (manual of self-help devices for the stroke pt.), *Up And Around* (booklet on activities of daily living), and *Stroke: Why Do They Behave That Way*, American Heart Association, 7320 Greenville Ave., Dallas, TX 75231.
"Physical Assessment—Part A: General Principles, Part B: Inspection, Part C: Palpation & Percussion, Part D: Auscultation." *NCP Guides #4:47, 48, 49, 50*, Nurseco, 1978.
"Stroke: The Double Crisis," by Glen McCormick and Margaret Williams. *American Journal of Nursing*, August 1979:1410–1411.
"Teaching Patients: General Suggestions." *NCP GUIDE #1:49*, 2nd. Ed., Nurseco, 1980.
"Teaching Patients: Specific Plan for Skills and Procedures." *NCP GUIDE #1:50*, 2nd. Ed., Nurseco, 1980.
"The Aged Patient: Remotivation." *NCP Guide #4:35*, Nurseco, 1978.
"The Aged Patient: Resocialization." *NCP Guide #3:34*, Nurseco, 1977.
"The Patient with Aphasia/Dysphasia." *NCP Guide #4:03*, Nurseco, 1978.
"The Patient with Cerebral-Vascular Accident (Acute Phase)." *NCP Guide #1:01*, 2nd. Ed., Nurseco, 1980.

The Patient with a Cholecystectomy

Definitions: A cholecystectomy is removal of the gallbladder; a choledochostomy is removal of stones from the common bile duct. If an obstruction is caused by a tumor, removal is accompanied by anastomosis of the bile duct stump to the intestinal tract—a choledochoduodenostomy or a choledochojejunostomy.

LONG TERM GOAL: The patient will recover successfully without preventable complications from biliary tract surgery and will return to usual roles in home, job, community after a normal convalescence.

General Considerations:

— **Signs and Symptoms** of acute cholecystitis: fever, leukocytosis, severe spasms of upper abdominal pain, anorexia, nausea, vomiting, distention, dark urine, clay-colored stools, jaundice and pruritis are common. In most cases gallstones (cholelithiasis) are present, causing obstruction, inflammation, edema and back-up of bile, depending on location of stones. Cholangiography confirms diagnosis.

— **Medical treatment** consists of attempts to dissolve the stone(s) with drugs, and to provide relief of symptoms with medications, nasogastric suction, parenteral therapy, antibiotics, and skin-soothing baths and lotions.

— Repeated attacks produce tissue scarring, nutritional deficiencies and liver damage; if medical treatment does not suffice, surgery is recommended (2 out of 3 cases) after the acute episode is controlled and the patient's condition is stabilized, if possible.

— **Nursing responsibilities** in the care of patients for biliary tract surgery are standard; refer to NCPG #2:44, "General Preoperative Nursing Care." In addition, the nurse explains about the drainage tubes that will be present and about the importance of turning, coughing, deep breathing and early ambulation—since these patients are more susceptible to pulmonary complications postop. Vitamin K is given for low prothrombin levels; blood transfusions may be needed; and carbohydrates are given orally or IV to build up glycogen stores in the liver.

Specific Considerations, Potential Patient Outcomes, and Nursing Actions:

1) General Abdominal Surgery Postop Measures

The patient maintains adequate cardio/pulmonary, elimination, musculoskeletal and other normal body functions; the patient is free of preventable complications of hemorrhage, infection, pneumonia, etc.:

— refer to NCPGs #2:41, 42, 43, "General Postoperative Nursing Care, Part A, Part B, Part C";

— record vital signs as ordered; measure & record I & O carefully & accurately; note color of urine & stools; check for re-establishment of voiding & elimination patterns;

— because of high incision & pain, vigorous turning, coughing & deep breathing exercises are needed Q2H; change position Q1-2H; dangle legs & ambulate gradually but firmly on schedule within the first 24 hrs.;

— place in low Fowler's position to facilitate drainage; encourage movement & exercises in bed; support abdomen with binder;

— give analgesics, sedatives, antibiotics, & other medications as ordered; observe for untoward reactions;

— check dressings closely & frequently for bleeding, especially first 8 hours.

2) Diet and Fluids	The patient maintains adequate fluid and electrolyte balance and is free of preventable imbalances; normal gastrointestinal function is restored and the patient tolerates solid foods in special diet: — monitor & record parenteral fluids & supplements; — keep NG tube patent, functioning; record color & amt. of drainage; give conscientious oral hygiene Q2H; when NG tube clamped, note pt.'s tolerance (nausea, vomiting, distention, bowel sounds) & report to MD; offer ice chips; after NG tube removed, give clear to full liquids as tolerated; then soft to regular low fat, high CHO, high Pro diet as ordered; — supplemental fat-soluble vitamins or a daily multivitamin is usually ordered; bile salts (oral adm. of Zanchol or Decholin Sodium) may be replaced to facilitate fat absorption; provide dietary consultation, assistance & instruction PRN.
3) Bile Drainage	Tissue edema at operative site subsides as bile is temporarily drained; normal biliary drainage internally is gradually restored: — keep T-tube, Penrose or drainage catheter unkinked & securely attached to straight tube & collection bag; avoid dependent loops & maintain prescribed height of bag to assure desired pressure level; — observe & record amt. & color of drainage; report persistent bleeding; obtain an order to irrigate, aspirate or clamp tube even for short periods; keep dressing & skin around suture line scrupulously clean, dry & free of irritating bile drainage; antibacterial skin protective ointments & skin barriers (ex. Stomahesive) should be used; anchor tube to dressing to prevent its pull on skin suture when pt. moves; — observe for signs of peritonitis resulting from bile leakage internally; report promptly fever, abdominal pain, distention, rigidity or untoward signs of change in pt.'s vital signs or status; explain to pt. & family all postop measures & cholangiography, lab work, etc.; — when ordered, tube will be clamped for 2-4 hr. periods around mealtime to observe pt.'s tolerance; note & report nausea, vomiting, chills, fever, increased pain or distention; reconnect tube to drainage bag PRN, otherwise clamping periods will be lengthened to 24, then 48 hrs.; if well tolerated, MD will remove tube & apply dry, sterile dressing to be changed PRN; observe stools & urine for reappearance of normal color; observe skin and sclerae for any indication of jaundice.

Discharge Planning and Teaching Objectives/Outcomes

1) (Patient/Family/Significant Other) Has written appointment, date and time for follow-up visit to surgeon.
2) States s/he knows what to expect re: length of convalescence (approx. six weeks), diet (as tolerated, but usually lower in fat) and care of operative site (soap and water cleansing; dry, sterile dressing). If taking medications home, knows what they are, indications, expected effects, dosage and administration.
3) Knows to call doctor for signs of illness, abdominal distention or pain, fever or breaking away of incision.

Recommended References
"General Preoperative Nursing Care," *NCP Guide* #2:44, 2nd Ed., Nurseco, 1980
"General Postoperative Nursing Care, Parts A, B and C," *NCP Guides* #2:41, 2:42, 2:43, 2nd Ed., Nurseco, 1980.

The Patient with Cirrhosis of the Liver

Definition: A chronic, progressive disease in which scar tissue replaces liver tissue causing degeneration of the liver, decreased functioning, and increased resistance to portal blood flow.

LONG TERM GOAL: The patient will maintain self within the limitations of prescribed medical regimen in order to reduce the progress of liver damage.

General Considerations:
— The **most common types** of hepatic cirrhosis are: (1) *Laennec's portal cirrhosis* (scar tissue develops in portal area) and (2) *postnecrotic* (following acute infections); the former type is more frequent than the latter.
— Laennec's cirrhosis **occurs** most frequently in persons (primarily men) over 50 years of age who have a history of long-term alcohol abuse.
— The exact **cause** of cirrhosis is not defined, but it is seen most often with chronic alcoholism and the resultant nutritional (protein) deficiency.
— In **early stages** of the disease, the patient will experience mild GI symptoms, fever, and liver enlargement; in **later stages,** chronic liver malfunction and obstruction of portal circulation create multiple imbalances and alterations in physiology.
— **Treatment** usually includes conservative measures (bed rest, diet, control of bleeding and symptoms, prevention of complications) in an effort to maintain as much liver function as possible and to retard progress of the disease.
— **Nursing responsibilities** include measures to help control bleeding (many of these patients enter the hospital because of bleeding varices), close monitoring of fluid and electrolyte status, ensuring compliance with medical regimen, and teaching patient to care for self adequately after discharge.

Specific Considerations, Potential Patient Outcomes, and Nursing Actions:

1) Control of Bleeding

The patient will adhere to prescribed regimen to stop hemorrhage; will maintain a patent airway; will experience no more than a moderate amount of anxiety:
— explain all procedures to pt. including rationale, expected discomforts, results; assess *how much* information pt. wants & provide only that amt.; be aware that giving information is an effective way to reduce anxiety but that giving too much may only increase it;
— assist with insertion of Sengstaken-Blakemore tube if used; provide pt. support during procedure;
— when tube is in place, ensure that it is taped so a tautness is kept on it in order to prevent it from slipping down into the main body of the stomach;

— label each lumen carefully & accurately as to amt. of pressure or volume in each & frequency of inflation/deflation; know that sufficient pressure must be given to retard the bleeding & that it must be released periodically to prevent necrosis of the tissue surrounding the tube; check Dr.'s orders on this & write the information clearly on the kardex;

— ensure proper functioning of suction equipment attached to tube; measure drainage carefully & chart;

— keep pt. NPO while tube is in place; if foods or fluid are given through the tube, give slowly in order to avoid regurgitation of the tube;

— provide emesis basin & wipes; keep a suction on hand & suction posterior pharynx PRN;

— know that a complication of tube placement is acute respiratory distress due to occlusion of airway by the balloon, and/or regurgitation of gastric contents into the lungs; if this should occur, cut tube lumens immediately; keep a pair of scissors taped in an obvious place at pt.'s bedside for such an emergency;

— observe for hematemesis, melena, & other signs of bleeding;

— take vital signs at least Q4H & PRN.

2) Fluid and Electrolytes

The patient is monitored for alterations in fluid and electrolyte balance:

— record I&O accurately; weigh pt. QD;

— check with Dr. re: daily amount of fluids allowed; if pt. on oral fluids, provide those within dietary restrictions, personal likes/dislikes;

— know normal values for serum electrolytes & liver function tests & compare to pt.'s values; if pt. wants to know, share this information with him, pointing out signs of positive change as they occur; refer to NCPGs #2:48, "Potassium Imbalance," & #s 3:48 & 3:49, "Fluids & Electrolytes";

— observe amt. & location of edema; chart daily & as changes occur;

— chart daily: presence & depth of jaundice of skin & sclera; color, odor & character of feces; color of urine.

3) Nutritional Alteration

The patient will ingest and adhere to prescribed diet in an effort to prevent further liver damage:

— know that adequate nutrition is often as important as meds. for these pts.; diet will usually be hi-protein, hi-caloric;

— explain rationale for diet to pt. & work with him to make meals as attractive & interesting as possible;

— provide frequent small meals with protein supplements, rather than three large meals;

— if ascites & edema are present, sodium will be restricted; check with Dr. re: using a salt substitute on tray; teach pt. to use other flavorings (e.g. lemon juice, oregano); refer to NCPG #3:44, "Diets: Low Sodium."

4) Skin Integrity

The patient will maintain skin integrity; will be free of skin breakdown, decubitus ulcer or infections; will experience relief of pruritis and skin discomfort:

— know that these pts. are prone to skin breakdown due to poor nutritional state, edema, muscle wasting, & immobility;

— turn Q2H & keep off back as much as possible;

— consider using an air mattress, sheepskin; refer to NCPG #4:42, "Decubitus Ulcer Care";
— provide ROM exercises PRN; check with Dr. as to which ones to use; refer to NCPG #1:47, "ROM Exercises";
— keep room cool & give antipruritic med. as ordered, in an effort to control pruritis;
— provide *gentle* rubbing, patting or stroking of skin; apply powder, talc or cornstarch; avoid soap; keep skin dry.

5) Rest and Comfort

The patient will obtain adequate oxygenation; will achieve an adequate rest-sleep pattern; will experience minimal emotional stress:
— know that SOB occurs often due to ascites; explain relationship to pt.; observe for changes in breathing, cyanosis;
— position pt. in a sitting position, supporting back & arms;
— keep supplies within easy reach of pt. so s/he will not have to struggle to get them;
— provide adequate oral hygiene PRN;
— turn at least Q2H; know that minimal movement may help decrease any nausea & vomiting.

6) Prevention of Complications

The patient will be monitored for early signs of hepatic encephalopathy, pulmonary congestion:
— know & observe for early signs of hepatic encephalopathy (including euphoria, inappropriate behavior, fatigue, irritability, restlessness, loss of judgement) and pulmonary congestion;
— observe & chart mental status 2 or 3 times daily; refer to NCPG #4:41, "Assessment of Mental Status";
— know & observe for additional signs of impending hepatic coma (nausea & vomiting, lo-grade fever, diarrhea, abdominal ache or pain); chart & report to Dr.

Discharge Planning and Teaching Objectives/Outcomes
1) (Patient/Family/Significant Other) Is aware that patient is susceptible to infection and knows preventive measures to carry out after discharge.
2) Understands that alcohol should be eliminated from diet and has community resources or referrals to this end (e.g. AA, social worker).
3) Can prepare menus within prescribed dietary restrictions.
4) Verbalizes an understanding of the relationship between rest, proper diet, and preservation of liver function.

Recommended References

"Controlling Chronic Liver Disease," by Morton J. Rodman, Ph.D. *RN*, February 1976:75–76, 79.

"Conquering Cirrhosis of the Liver & A Dangerous Complication," by Patricia O. Dolan, RN, MS and Harry L. Green II, MD. *Nursing 76*, November 1976:44–53.

"Decubitis Ulcer Care: Prevention and Treatment," *NCP Guide #4:42*, Nurseco, 1979.

"Diets: Low Sodium," *NCP Guide #3:44*, Nurseco, 1977.

"Fluids & Electrolytes, Part A: Fluids," "Part B: Electrolytes," *NCP Guides #3:48 & 49*, Nurseco, 1977.

"How to Salvage a Bleeding Cirrhosis Patient," by Francis L. Martin, RN, MS. *RN*, January 1980:59–65.

"Potassium Imbalance," *NCP Guide #2:48*, 2nd ed., Nurseco, 1980.

"Range of Motion Exercises," *NCP Guide #1:47*.

"Realistic Nursing Goals In Terminal Cirrhosis," *Nursing 78*, June 1978:43–47.

"Symposium on Diseases of the Liver," Boyer, Carol A. and Oehlberg, Susan M., Guest Editors. *Nursing Clinics of North America*, June 1977:257–356.

The Patient with a Colostomy

Definition:　Colostomy is a surgically constructed bowel outlet on the abdomen, using some portion of the large intestine.

LONG TERM GOAL:　The patient will recover from a successful colostomy without preventable complications returning to optimum health possible and usual roles in home, job, community after a normal convalescence; the patient will accept and cope realistically and adaptively to an altered body image and loss of normal elimination function.

General Considerations:
- **Indications** include: Hirschsprung's disease, diverticulitis, cancer, bowel perforation, obstruction or trauma, radiation enteritis.
- Colostomy may be **temporary** or **permanent**. The latter involves complete removal of the colon and rectum (proctocolectomy) and abdomino-perineal resection, usually. If the patient's condition and disease warrants, a temporary colostomy will be closed and the bowel re-anastomosed after it has healed. Closure may be done anytime from two months to a year, depending on the patient's condition.
- **Nursing responsibilities** include assessment, physical preparation of the patient and the bowel, plus psychological and emotional preparation of the patient (when time permits, if the operation is not an emergency).
- **Assessment** includes finding out:
  - whether the colostomy is to be temporary or permanent;
  - whether an abdominal-perineal resection and proctectomy will be done;
  - whether the patient has cancer and to what extent;
  - whether the patient will have chemotherapy and/or radiation postoperatively;
  - what the site of the colostomy will be (ascending, transverse, or descending colon);
  - whether the surgeon has thoroughly discussed the proposed operation with the patient and family; and
  - whether the patient and family really understands what is to be done.
- **Physical preparation of the patient** includes: obtaining operative and anesthesia consents, skin prep, preoperative sedation, preoperative assessment and teaching. Refer to NCPG #2:44, "General Preoperative Nursing Care."
- **Preparation of the bowel** to empty it, decompress it and reduce its bacteria includes:
  - low residue diet four days pre-op, clear liquids day before surgery, NPO after midnight and nasogastric intubation morning of surgery;
  - purgatives and cleansing enemas (tap water or saline) are given 1-4 days before scheduled operation; and
  - sulfa drugs or broad-spectrum antibiotics for two days pre-op.

— **Psychological and emotional preparation of the patient** includes:
  — an assessment of the level of acceptance (or the point in the grieving process) regarding the proposed operation and its implications for both patient and family;
  — encouragement of patient/family/significant other to express fears freely (Common and normal fears include those of dying, of pain, of cancer and its extent, of the success of surgery, of the changes in body appearance and function, of the loss of sexual interest, appeal and performance, of rejection of partner, family and friends, of a lengthy and costly hospitalization and of loss of independence/control.);
  — provision of explanations & clear, honest, direct answers to patient/family questions, resolving misconceptions & conflicting information;
  — reassurance & emotional support without raising false hopes or misleading patient (Sometimes this can best be provided by an enterostomal therapist or a successfully rehabilitated, mature, responsible colostomate.).

Specific Considerations, Potential Patient Outcomes, and Nursing Actions:

1) General Abdominal Surgery Postop Measures

The patient maintains adequate cardio/pulmonary, musculoskeletal and renal functions; the patient is free of preventable complications of hemorrhage, infection, pneumonia and stomal damage; the patient is carefully monitored and maintains fluid and electrolyte balance:
  — refer to NCPG's #2:41, 42, 43, "General Postoperative Nursing Care, Parts A, B, C";
  — monitor & record vital signs, CVP readings as ordered;
  — monitor administration of parenteral fluids, electrolytes & vitamin supplements; refer to NCPG #2:46, "Intravenous Therapy: General Principles,"NCPG #3:48 & #3:49, "Fluids & Electrolytes, Part A & Part B";
  — record intake & output accurately; check urine output hourly, noting specific gravity; refer to NCPG #2:39, "Catheters: Indwelling Urinary";
  — watch for signs of electrolyte imbalance; check lab reports; see NCPG #2:48, "Potassium Imbalance";
  — turn, cough & deep breathe pt. Q2H; have pt. exercise arms & legs between position changes; position for comfort & to avoid tension on operative site; provide binder for abdominal support;
  — keep NG tube functioning & patent until tube is removed; record amt. & color of drainage; measure & record amt. used for irrigating NG tube; give oral hygiene Q2H;
  — administer analgesics, sedatives, antibiotics as ordered.

2) Perineal Wound Care

The patient's perineal wound will drain, be kept clean and heal without infection:
  — change or reinforce dressing as necessary to keep clean & dry;
  — note & record color, odor & amount of drainage;
  — when permitted, give sitz baths twice or more daily.

3) Abdominal Would Care

The patient's abdominal wound will drain, be kept clean and heal without infection:
  — change or reinforce dressing as necessary;

— note color, odor, & amt. of drainage;
— keep surrounding skin area clean, dry & protected from irritants.

4) Nutrition

The patient will resume special diet as tolerated:
— when peristalsis returns, NG tube is clamped & clear liquids are given (about 30 ml. hourly); observe for signs of abdominal distention, pain, nausea & vomiting; reconnect tube to suction if signs occur;
— at 4 hr. intervals, unclamp NG tube to measure amt. of residual gastric content; if less than prescribed amt., then NG tube will be ordered removed;
— gradually resume liquid, then soft, then regular consistency bland, low residue foods; note pt.'s tolerance & intake;
— ask pt. to chew food slowly with mouth closed to reduce air intake & gas pains; refrain from using a drinking straw; teach patient to avoid gas-forming foods such as beans, cauliflower, cabbage, onions, cucumbers, carbonated drinks, etc.

5) Colostomy
   Care

The patient will eliminate fecal discharge through colostomy via irrigations or collection bag; the peristomal skin will be protected from irritation and infection; the patient will learn self-care of colostomy:
— know that during the immediate postop period, the exposed bowel is covered with ointment-impregnated gauze & abdominal pads which are to be changed PRN to prevent contamination of adjacent sutures;
— after the bowel is opened by the surgeon, a temporary collection bag is applied; it is emptied when 1/3 full & changed when loose or leaking; teach pt. to do this when sitting on the toilet; rinse & dry bag with toilet tissue before reclamping; use bag & room deodorants to prevent pt. embarrassment; teach appliance change & skin care to pt.; refer to NCPG #1:43, "Basic Principles for Changing a Temporary or Permanent Appliance";
— observe & record color, odor & amt. of fecal drainage; observe & report stomal retraction or protrusion, peristomal irritation & infection; tell pt. that stoma will shrink in size over the next several weeks as healing occurs & initial swelling subsides; stress that because of this, it is necessary to measure stoma each time appliance is changed in order to protect the surrounding skin from irritating leakage;
— know that colostomy discharge *may* be regulated by diet, laxatives, suppositories and/or irrigation (still quite common), but regularity is also dependent upon the location of the colostomy, fluid intake, exercise, emotional influences & the pt.'s physical & psychological condition; don't promise a pt. "regularity" as it may not be possible;
— if irrigations are ordered, check with procedure manual & an experienced nurse as they should be done with smoothness, efficiency & care to foster a positive attitude in the pt.;
— consult nearest Enterostomal Therapist for information & help with pt.

6) Psychosocial
   Adjustment

The patient will adapt realistically to an altered body image and self-concept; the patient will cope effectively with loss of normal body elimination, accepting colostomy and caring for it with confidence; the family expresses understanding and acceptance of the patient's altered condition and provides emotional support to the patient:

— be sensitive to behavioral cues: depression, tears, silence, apathy; refusal to cooperate may indicate feelings of anger, grief, shame, disgust, embarrassment, loss of self-esteem associated with the shocking reality of the operation (& possibly a diagnosis of cancer); refer to NCPG #1:31, "Responses to Loss; the Grief and Mourning Process";

— needs of pt. include being listened to, being accepted & cared about, being understood as having normal feelings & regaining self-control; be available; be a good listener; be matter-of-fact, yet sympathetic; be calm & confident, yet concerned;

— remember the emotional impact may be as great for pts. with a temporary colostomy as for pts. with a permanent colostomy; closure can't be predicted & do not over-emphasize the "temporary" nature of the colostomy;

— see NCP Guides on specific behaviors presented by pt. (#'s1:20-33); discuss pt.'s responses with pt., family & nursing staff; work together toward a realistic plan of care & put approaches on written nursing care plan;

— arrange to have a successfully rehabilitated colostomate and/or an enterostomal therapist visit pt.;

— encourage pt. to look at & touch stoma; refer to NCPG #2:29, "The Patient Experiencing a Body Image Disturbance";

— provide pt./family/significant other with informational booklets from the American Cancer Society, the United Ostomy Association, or other sources as deemed appropriate; see recommended references;

— recognize intimacy as a valued need & encourage open discussions between pt. & partner; provide information & correct misconceptions.

Discharge Planning and Teaching Objectives/Outcomes

1) (Patient/Family/Significant Other) States s/he knows basic facts and instructions re: diet, exercise (restriction of heavy lifting), medications (dosage, purpose, side effects to be reported) and return to usual activities.
2) Can describe the type of surgery and kind of stoma s/he has; demonstrates correct, safe, confident care of colostomy and appliance change;
3) Knows to report promptly to physician complications, abdominal cramps, repeated vomiting, diarrhea, constipation, pain, fever or other illness.
4) Knows how to handle *minor* temporary episodes of constipation, diarrhea and peristomal skin irritation.
5) Has an identification wallet card listing medications, routine of colostomy care, the name and phone number of physician, and the next of kin to be notified in case of an accident.
6) Has at least two weeks' colostomy supplies and the name and address of local supplier for additional needs.
7) Has been evaluated for assistance (financial, vocational, social service disability, homemaker and home health care) and has received appropriate referrals.
8) Has the name and phone number of nearest enterostomal therapist and/or community health nurse.

9) Has received literature and information appropriate to needs and concerns; knows how to contact local ostomy association for further support services.

10) Has received the address of The United Ostomy Assn., Inc., 2001 Beverly Blvd., Los Angeles, CA 90057.

Recommended References

"A New Ball Game For Colostomy Patients," by Charlotte Isler. *RN*, September 1977:52, 53.

"Basic Principles for Changing a Temporary or Permanent Appliance." *NCP Guide* #1:43, 2nd Ed., Nurseco, 1980.

Care of Your Colostomy (a source book of information for patients). American Cancer Society, 219 E. 42nd St., New York, NY 10017.

"Catheters: Indwelling Urethral." *NCP Guide* #2:39, 2nd Ed., Nurseco, 1980.

Colostomies—A Guide (English, French, Spanish or Chinese). United Ostomy Assn., 2001 Beverly Blvd., Los Angeles, CA 90057.

"Colostomy Irrigation Yes or No?", by Rosemary Watt. *American Journal of Nursing*, March 1977:442–444.

"Fluids & Electrolytes, Part A: Fluids, Part B: Electrolytes." *NCP Guides* #3:48 & #3:49, Nurseco, 1977.

"General Postoperative Nursing Care, Part A, Part B, Part C." *NCP Guides* #2:41, #2:42, #2:43, 2nd Ed., Nurseco, 1980.

"General Preoperative Nursing Care." *NCP Guide* #2:44, 2nd Ed., Nurseco, 1980.

"Intravenous Therapy: General Principles." *NCP Guide* #2:46, 2nd Ed., Nurseco, 1980.

"Loop Transverse Colostomy," by Debra Broadwell and Suzanne Sorrells. *American Journal of Nursing*, June 1978;1029–1031.

"Potassium Imbalance." *NCP Guide* #2:48, 2nd Ed., Nurseco, 1980.

"Responses to Loss: the Grief and Mourning Process." *NCP Guide* #1:31, 2nd Ed., Nurseco, 1980.

"Teaching Patients: General Suggestions." *NCP Guide* #1:49, 2nd Ed., Nurseco, 1980.

"Teaching Patients: Specific Plan for Skills and Procedures." *NCP Guide* #1:50, 2nd Ed., Nurseco, 1980.

"The Patient Experiencing a Body Image Disturbance." *NCP Guide* #2:29, 2nd Ed., Nurseco, 1980.

The Patient with Congestive Heart Failure:
Chronic or Post Emergency Phase

Definition: Circulatory congestion related to inadequate cardiac output as a result of decreased force and efficiency of myocardial contraction.

LONG TERM GOAL: The patient will reach optimum level of functioning within the limits of cardiac condition; the patient states s/he understands and feels able to follow a therapeutic regimen designed to prevent complications and recurrences and to maximize rehabilitation gains.

General Considerations:
— **Backward theory of CHF:** When the heart ventricles cannot accommodate the blood volume it receives, a back-up occurs . . . in the lungs (left-sided failure) and/or . . . in the systemic blood vessels (right-sided failure). While either side of the heart may fail separately, usually both sides are involved and the patient is treated accordingly.
— **Treatment aim:** To decrease the work of the heart by reducing circulating blood volume and edema; **treatment plan includes:** rest, digitalization, diuretics, diet, and symptomatic relief measures.
— During the **acute phase** of CHF, patients should be monitored closely and receive intensive nursing and medical care in CCUs. Following the critical stage, when the patient's condition has stabilized, s/he is transferred to Cardiac Rehabilitation Units (CRUs) or intermediate nursing units for continuing treatment, education, rehabilitative measures and preparation for discharge to home or convalescent hospital. Refer to Nursing Care Planning Guide #2:11, "The Patient with Congestive Heart Failure: Acute Phase," for further information about CHF and relevant nursing care.

Specific Considerations, Potential Patient Outcomes, and Nursing Actions:
1) Rest and Comfort

The patient will experience decreased episodes of dyspnea, angina and dysrythmias as well as lessened anxiety and tension; the work load of the heart will be reduced thereby decreasing the need for oxygen to meet the body's lessened metabolic demands:
— know that, depending on pt.'s functional classification, doctor will order specific type of bed or chair rest with specific ADL permitted & amt. of assistance to be provided; be certain that all nursing care personnel are clear & consistent in implementing this;
— position pt. in mid or high Fowler's; support with pillows; place footboard & overbed table in position to maintain pt. for easier breathing;
— prevent pressure areas with good skin care and frequent position changes; use sheepskin, cushions & other protection devices; refer to NCPG #4:42, "Decubitus Ulcer Care: Prevention and Treatment";

— provide a cool, well-ventilated quiet room with limited visitors; do not permit smoking or noisy conversations in room;

— provide rest periods between meals & care; block incoming phone calls at this time;

— prevent constipation & straining at defecation with ordered laxatives, enemas, fluid intake, use of commode or bathroom when permitted;

— administer Morphine or other analgesic as ordered for pain, apprehension;

— give sedatives & hypnotics to reduce restlessness & induce short sleeping periods;

— have nitroglycerine tabs. accessible PRN;

— teach & give deep breathing & passive leg exercises QID;

— wrap legs with elastic bandages from heel to groin, rewrap Q6H & PRN;

— employ relaxation measures, i.e. soft music, a comforting visitor, reading to pt., unhurried nursing care, short & slow walks with rest stops, when permitted;

— if pt. is able to talk without increasing dyspnea, encourage him to talk with you, to express concerns & fears; common ones include fear of dying, of invalidism, of dependency, of unknown future; allow pt. to ask questions; provide information to both pt. & family;

— emphasize belief that critical period is past, that gaining strength, increasing activity tolerance & learning to care for self is objective now;

— observe or note report of exercise tolerance studies; consult with MD & physical therapist for exercise schedule & ADL to implement.

2) Nutrition, Fluids and Electrolytes

Edema will be lessened; abdominal distention and pressure on diaphragm will be minimized; the patient will participate in a weight loss program through a nutritious diet that is accepted and understood:

— offer attractive, small frequent feedings of soft, bland, low Na, low caloric, low residue, low fat, non-gas forming foods; consider likes & dislikes; have dietician see pt. PRN; teach pt./family about dietary needs & requirements after discharge; refer to NCPG #3:44, "Diets: Low Sodium," and #3:43, "Diets: Fat-Controlled, Low Cholesterol";

— after determining type of diuretic being given (potassium-sparing or not), obtain sodium substitutes and other desired food flavorings (lemon, vinegar, almond & vanilla) to enhance palatibility of bland diet;

— provide fluids as ordered, especially those high in potassium (if needed); avoid carbonated or caffeinated beverages, refrain from having drinks too hot or too cold;

— provide vitamin & mineral supplements as ordered;

— anorexia, nausea & vomiting are common; consider digitalis or diuretic toxicity as well as mineral depletion; observe & report other signs & symptoms; refer to NCPG #2:48, "Potassium Imbalance."

3) Digitalization   The patient's heart beat will be slowed, strengthened and steadied; cardiac output will be increased:
    — record & administer digitalis preparations as prescribed; check apical & radial pulses (rate, rhythm, & volume) as ordered;
    — watch closely for toxic effects (nausea, diarrhea, pulse slowness or irregularities, "yellow" vision, etc.) & report to Dr. promptly;
    — refer to NCPG #2:37, "Drugs: Cardiac."

4) Diuretics &   Sodium excretion will be increased; tissue fluid retention will be lessened:
   Control of   — record weight daily on same scale in same amt. of clothing;
   Edema   — keep careful I & O record, estimating perspiration;
    — record degree of pitting edema (sacral & pedal);
    — elevate extremities, support legs; provide good skin care;
    — observe & report signs of drug toxicity & mineral depletion (muscle cramps, headaches, dizziness, skin rashes, etc.) especially potassium loss (lassitude, mental confusion, decreased urinary output); check serum potassium level; see NCPG #2:48, "Potassium Imbalance";
    — give potassium supplements if ordered.

5) Prevention of   The patient will be free of preventable complications or have them recognized and controlled promptly and competently:
   Complications   — observe for signs of orthopnea & paroxysmal nocturnal dyspnea (sudden, severe shortness of breath about 2 hours after going to bed);
    — note cyanosis, restlessness, anxious behavior, rapid & thready pulse, struggle to sit or stand in order to breathe;
    — check blood gas levels, vital signs as frequently as condition warrants;
    — observe for signs of pulmonary edema (gurgling respirations, bloody & frothy sputum, profuse sweating, constant coughing, acute distress); refer to NCPG #2:21, "The Patient with Pulmonary Edema";
    — start O_2; notify doctor STAT, give Morphine & bronchial dilators according to emergency protocols; have available cardiac emergency drugs, equipment, IV supplies;
    — note onset of ascites and/or pleural effusion; have centesis trays available.

Discharge Planning and Teaching Objectives/Outcomes

1) (Patient/Family/Significant Other) Can state in own words the basic facts of CHF, signs and symptoms, treatment and prevention of complications. Has received and read AHA leaflet on subject.

2) Has general outline of activity permitted; knows to avoid smokers, smoky environments and those with colds or other illnesses.

3) Has an appointment for follow-up medical care.

4) Has received and read written instructions re: medications, dosage, administration, desired effects and untoward or toxic symptoms to be reported promptly to doctor.

5) Has received, read and indicates s/he understands written dietary instructions; can plan a typical day's menu and tell what is permitted or disallowed on diet; knows how to find out the sodium content in local water supply and whether or not s/he should drink bottled water; knows whether or not s/he needs to purchase low sodium food products.

6) Has been evaluated for social and financial assistance, and, if needed, appropriate referrals have been made to state or local agencies.

7) Has at least one community health resource person's name and number (besides doctor) in order to get additional help and information; knows about the counseling and information services available at most local heart associations.

8) Has an identification card for wallet with name and address, next of kin's name, address and phone number, doctor's name and phone number, the diagnosis, medications and dosage and allergies (if any); knows how s/he can obtain a small portable O_2 tank and mask for emergency use at home.

Recommended References

"Decubitus Ulcer Care: Prevention and Treatment." *NCP Guide* #4:42, Nurseco, 1978.

"Diets: Fat Controlled, Low Cholesterol." *NCP Guide* #3:43, Nurseco, 1977.

"Diets: Low Sodium." *NCP Guide* #3:44, Nurseco, 1977.

"Drugs: Cardiac." *NCP Guide* #2:37, 2nd Ed., Nurseco, 1980.

Facts About Congestive Heart Failure. American Heart Association, 7320 Greenville Ave., Dallas, TX 75231.

"Heart Failure in the MI Patient," by Gloria Tanner. *American Journal of Nursing*, February 1977:230–234.

"Potassium Imbalance." *NCP Guide* #2:48, 2nd Ed., Nurseco, 1980.

"The Patient with Congestive Heart Failure: Acute Phase." *NCP Guide* #2:11, 2nd Ed., Nurseco, 1980.

The Patient with Diabetes

Definition: Diabetes mellitus is a chronic, metabolic disorder which affects the body's ability to manufacture and/or utilize insulin (the hormone produced by the beta cells of the pancreas).

LONG TERM GOAL: The patient will reach and maintain the optimum level of performance possible, living within the limits of the disease and treatment regimen, preventing as much as possible the pathological changes and complications of diabetes; the patient will accept and integrate successfully the diabetic lifestyle into self-concept and will achieve self-confident control; the patient will resume normal home, family, community roles with necessary adaptation.

General Considerations:
— **Incidence:** directly affects 10 million Americans (over 50 million affected indirectly via family ties); incidence increasing yearly; probability increases with age and obesity; disease found more commonly in women, in non-whites, in those with yearly incomes of under $5000.
— **Types: Juvenile**—onset before 39 years of age, usually insulin-dependent, a virus has been implicated as a possible causal factor; **Mature**—onset in later years, often controlled by diet alone or with oral med., causal factors related to obesity and heredity. **Diagnosis** includes a fasting blood sugar, 2 Hr. Post-Prandial, and a thorough physical & history.
— **Signs and Symptoms:** Frequent urination (polyuria), excessive thirst (polydipsia), fatigue, loss of weight associated with excessive hunger (polyphagia), and chronic infections slow to heal. Peripheral neuropathy (diminished sensations) is common.
— **Treatment** aims: to control symptoms and to prevent or control complications associated with metabolic, neurologic, and cardiovascular consequences of the disease. **Education** of the patient and family is the keystone of quality care, whether the patient is newly diagnosed, or is a re-admission for surgery, illness, injury or associated complication.
— **Nursing responsibilities** (whether hospital staff, metabolic clinic, home health or occupational RN) involve assessment, education, counseling and assisting the patient and family to accept and cope effectively in the long-term management of this lifetime condition. After consulting with the physician re: the therapeutic regimen or prescribed diet, drugs, exercise and follow-up care, the nurse should interview the patient and family to determine what they know, what they need to know, and what their expectations are regarding hospitalization, treatment and care after discharge. In collaboration with them, establish objectives and plans for what should be taught, when and by whom. Obtain and review educational materials for them, which will be relevant and useful. Suggested teaching outcomes are given below.

Specific Considerations, Potential Patient Outcomes, and Nursing Actions:
1) Nutrition   The patient establishes and maintains ideal body weight and proper nutrition; the patient eats all food at proper times and does not eat between meal snacks, except as prescribed; the patient is able to meet dietary requirements in a liquid form whenever s/he is unable to chew, take solid foods, has missed or failed to finish a complete meal:

— give all meals & snacks on time; encourage full consumption; record & measure amounts left & give replacement carbohydrate feeding;

— administer vitamin & mineral supplements as ordered;

— see NCPG #1:36, "General Dietary Principles for the Diabetic," & NCPG #1:37, "Liquid Diet Substitutes for the Diabetic"; teach pt. & family about dietary planning or refer to teaching dietician for this.

2) Medications   The patient receives insulin or oral hypoglycemics as ordered; the patient knows about the different types of insulin, how to store and prepare for an injection; how to give own injections correctly, rotating sites according to a plan, and how to care for equipment safely:

— see NCPG #1:38, "Properties of Insulin Preparations"; teach pt. & family about insulin, its storage & handling, activity & effects;

— teach pt. & at least one family member to administer insulin correctly, safely & satisfactorily;

— teach pt. & family the factors that increase insulin need (trauma, infection, fever, exposure to cold, the adrenal hormones-catecholamines increased by stress & tension) & to avoid these factors when possible; if these influences are unavoidable, then to seek prompt medical advice;

— teach the importance & method of site rotation & provide a suitable chart for recording sites used with dates.

3) Exercise   The patient maintains a normal activity level for age to provide a balance for insulin and diet being given; the patient demonstrates the knowledge that exercise is an important part of treatment by being physically active on a daily basis:

— teach pt. that regular physical exercise done at least three times a week for 20 min. each time has the following benefits: *decreases* BP, body weight, appetite, tension, triglycerides and need for some insulin; (exercise) *increases* stamina, self-confidence and work performance;

— teach pt. to prepare for exercise by adjusting medication & food; have pt. be prepared (carry on person) with some form of quick acting sugar (jelly beans, Life Savers, Cake Mate Decorating Jell) in case of need;

— see recommended references for book on sports & exercise.

4) Prevention of Complications   The patient knows the common complications of diabetes (arteriosclerosis, chronic infections, eye trouble, neuritis, heart disease, kidney disease) and most of the early warning signs to report to his doctor; the patient and family can describe the difference between insulin reaction and ketoacidosis, can tell what to do for each situation; the patient and family demonstrate knowledge of good oral hygiene, proper skin and foot care and what to do for illness:

— know that the *first step* to preventing complications is *assessment* of the possibilities and recognition of the importance of the pt. having informed, self-confident control of his disease;

— hold frequent *conferences* with physician, dietician, social worker & other staff members to discuss pt.'s progress, to exchange suggestions & observations, to coordinate the treatment plan & teaching;

— *teach pt.* & *family* about *ketoacidosis* & *hypoglycemia*; refer to NCPG #1:35;

— evaluate pt.'s foot care needs; demonstrate proper *foot care* & supervise return demonstrations; see NCPG #1:39:

— know that glucose in the epidermis of diabetic pts. predisposes to *skin infections*; observe & report skin lesions; prevent chafing & irritation caused by perspiration by powdering skin surfaces & by teaching pt. to wear loose-fitting cotton garments next to skin;

— observe & report lesions of mouth, *gum and teeth conditions*; teach & supervise proper dental hygiene (including use of dental floss & disclosing tablets); refer to dentist PRN & follow-up to ensure this is done;

— know that blurred vision can result from changed glucose levels and insulin dosages: cataracts, glaucoma & retinopathy are also common; refer for *opthalmology evaluation* after condition stabilizes for two months & thereafter on a regular basis as recommended by progress of disease;

— check pt.'s *weight and BP* regularly; assess for weight gain, edema, gradual hypertension, anginal pains & report accordingly;

— assess for *peripheral vascular disease*; check pedal pulses, ulcerations & infections of feet & legs; note presence of intermittent claudication (leg pain only while walking);

— assess for *peripheral neuropathy*; note impaired sensation of feet & fingers; teach pt. caution while cooking, lighting matches, smoking, using heating appliances, being around extreme sources of heat or cold;

— observe & check for itching or burning on *urination*, diminished output, increased specific gravity, flank pain, urgency, frequency, dysuria, pneumaturia (bubbly voided urine due to action of bacteria upon glucose in urine); record & report all abnormal signs & symptoms; teach pt. & family to do this after discharge;

— remind pt. never to take patent or non-prescribed medicines (which may contain high amts. of sugar in flavoring or additives) unless their doctor knows & gives approval;

— teach pt. & family what to do in case of *minor short-term illness* (cold or flu, etc.):

    (1) *take insulin* as regularly prescribed (or regularly prescribed oral hypoglycemics, if tolerated) unless & until s/he can reach doctor;

    (2) go to bed & keep warm;

    (3) take fluids as tolerated every hour & keep a record of what taken & how much;

    (4) if s/he can't take solid foods, replace usual diet with semi-liquid carbohydrates (same number of grams); refer to NCPG #1:37, "Liquid Diet Substitutes for the Diabetic";

(5) test urine for sugar & acetone *at least* every four hours & keep a record of results;

(6) be in touch with doctor by phone, so s/he can monitor progress; if illness lasts more than 48 hours, or if symptoms grow worse, *see* doctor; notify doctor immediately for vomiting or diarrhea, because they upset the fluid & electrolyte balance quickly & reduce the blood sugar & insulin requirements; *remember* infection, fever & stress increase the need for insulin even if pt. can't eat normally, so insulin must be taken when ill;

— provide pt. with ID card for wallet indicating: doctor's name & address, types of medication being taken & how much, next of kin to be notified in emergency, & other pertinent information; an ID bracelet is more visible & quickly noticed, so help pt. arrange for getting one;

— urge pt. to visit doctor or clinic at least two months prior to taking an extended trip (especially outside country), so that minor health problems can be detected & corrected, so that immunization reactions have completed their course, so that adequate plans & precautions are considered; see recommended references for additional info; have pt. assemble all diabetic supplies & doctor's statement in "carry-on" hand luggage; tell pt. s/he can obtain additional info from: The International Diabetes Foundation, 3-6 Alfred Place, London, WCIE, 7EE, England.

5) Urine Testing   The patient will assess control daily by testing urine correctly and keeping records; the patient and at least one family member or friend will demonstrate the two-drop Clinitest method and the Acetest:

— teach pt. an appropriate method of testing urine after considering pt. needs & medications, advantages & disadvantages of products, & physician preference; refer to NCPG #1:50, "Teaching Patients—Skills and Procedures";

— explain reasons for not touching tablets or testing paper with fingers;

— know that medications & vitamins may affect results (ex. Vit. C & levodopa cause false negatives with Tes-Tape; Keflin, Aspirin & Vit. C cause false positives with Clinitests) so if pt. is taking drugs other than insulin, discuss appropriate testing material with pharmacist & physician;

— although research results are controversial, know that it is probably best to use a second, freshly voided specimen following a previous emptying of bladder; teach pt. reasons for doing so;

— know that percentage of sugar has differing "plus" meanings on various products so *record results in percentages only* & name the test used; teach the pt. & other staff to do so, as consistency is essential for correctly & effectively regulating insulin dosage; provide record form for listing results (including one for taking home);

— know that if pt. has over 2% sugar (a bright orange "pass through" phenomenon, when glycosuria is too high to react accurately), you should use & teach pt. the *"2 drop test"* (2 drops urine with 10 drops water) to further determine correct percentage of sugar, but you must *use a different color chart*;

— for visually impaired pts., teach the "touch test" (add baking soda to urine in a test tube, cover with a finger cot, feel the inflation caused by gaseous expansion showing presence of sugar) or use Mega-Diastix;

— for nursing mothers and pregnant women in third trimester, use an enzyme test (Tes-Tape, Diastix) to check for *glyco*suria because Clinitest will be positive for *lactose* in urine;

— for older persons, know that renal threshold for glucose rises with age, so pt. may be hyperglycemic without glycosuria, therefore, postprandial blood sugars may be needed.

6) Psychosocial Adjustment

The patient will demonstrate a productive, self-reliant adjustment to diabetic condition and management; the patient (and family) will express feelings of acceptance, self-confidence and relief of fear concerning condition:

— see NCPG #1:44, "Suggestions for Interviewing"; consult both pt. & family for assistance in planning, implementing & evaluating teaching program; refer to NCPG #1:49, "Teaching Patients: General Suggestions";

— observe family relationships to estimate degree of support available to pt. after discharge; consider enlisting the aid of a close friend PRN;

— provide pt. & family with address & phone number of local diabetes assn; encourage them to attend monthly lecture series & to participate in self-help groups; give them pamphlets to take home for future reference;

— know & be informed about diabetes-related sexual & reproductive malfunctions which may occur & which doubtlessly concern pt.; see recommended references; provide sound explanations with sympathetic counseling to alleviate anxiety associated with problem;

— know that emotional upsets & tension increase need for insulin; attempt to determine & alleviate causes of stress or help pt. to cope more effectively; provide opportunities for pt./family to express feelings, concerns, frustrations & annoyances;

— assess need for convalescent hospital or home health care assistance & make appropriate referrals.

Discharge Planning and Teaching Objectives/Outcomes

1) (Patient/Family/Significant Other) Can answer questions: What is diabetes, what are the common symptoms, treatment and expectations for its control? Has received at least one current pamphlet on diabetes and a written sheet of instructions regarding special aspects of condition.
2) Can test urine properly for sugar and acetone; knows how to keep an accurate record.
3) Can tell about types of insulin, how to store and handle it correctly; can give own injections accurately and safely, rotating sites according to a plan and caring for equipment without contamination.
4) Can state the differing symptoms and signs of hypoglycemia and ketoacidosis; knows exactly what to do for each situation.
5) Maintains a blood glucose of 80-200 mg.%; maintains a negative urine and acetone level.
6) Has a printed sheet of dietary instructions and sample menus. Can understand, accept and help plan a well-balanced meal consistent with prescribed grams of protein, carbohydrate, fat and calories needed to maintain ideal weight. Knows the general dietary rules of food measurement and preparation. Can list the foods allowed and those to avoid.

7) Can describe the meaning and importance of good personal health habits, including regular, moderate exercise; daily care of teeth, skin and feet; adequate rest and sleep; regular medical check-ups (including opthamologist and dentist).

8) Knows the common complications of diabetes (arteriosclerosis, chronic infections, eye trouble, skin lesions, neuritis, heart disease, kidney ailments) and the early warning signs to report to a doctor.

9) Has an identification card in wallet, which includes the name, address and phone number of next of kin, of physician, of self, as well as the names and dosages of medications, and what to do for an insulin reaction.

10) Knows the name and address of the American Diabetes Association and its local chapter. Is aware of the services available and knows of the availability of community health services in the home if necessary or desirable.

Recommended References

"Better Use of Resources Equals Better Health for Diabetics," by June Isaf and Maria Alogna. *American Journal of Nursing*, November 1977:1792–1795.

"Deliver Facts To Help Diabetics Plan Parenthood," by Catherine Garofano. *Nursing 77*, April 1977:13–16.

Diabetes Care, Diabetes Forecast, and other current literature. American Diabetes Association, 600 Fifth Ave., New York, NY 10020.

"Diagnosis and Management of Diabetes in the Elderly," by Charlotte Eliopoulos. *American Journal of Nursing*, May 1978:884–887.

"Differentiating Hypoglycemia and Ketoacidosis," *NCP Guide* #1:35, 2nd. Ed., Nurseco, 1980.

Education and Management of the Patient with Diabetes. Ames Co., Div. Miles Laboratories, Inc., P O Box 70, Elkhart, IN 46515.

"General Dietary Principles for the Diabetic," *NCP Guide* #1:36, 2nd. Ed., Nurseco, 1980.

"Liquid Diet Substitutes for the Diabetic," *NCP Guide* #1:37, 2nd. Ed., Nurseco, 1980.

Managing Diabetics Properly. Nursing 78 Books, Intermed Communications, Inc., Horsham, PA 19044.

Managing Your Diabetes, by Jean Ranch and Mae McWeeny. Abbot-Northwestern Hospital, Inc., 1978. (from Minneapolis Med. Center Publications Office, 810 E. 27th St., Minn., MN 55407).

"Properties of Insulin Preparations," *NCP Guide* #1:38, 2nd. Ed., Nurseco, 1980.

"Recommended Care of the Feet for Diabetics," *NCP Guide* #1:39, 2nd. Ed., Nurseco, 1980.

"Reporting Urine Test Results: Switch from + to %," by Dorothy Lundin. *American Journal of Nursing*, May 1978:878,879.

"Suggestions for Interviewing," *NCP Guide* #1:44, 2nd. Ed., Nurseco, 1980.

"Teaching Patients: General Suggestions," *NCP Guide* #1:49, 2nd. Ed., Nurseco, 1980.

"Teaching Patients: Specific Plan for Skills and Procedures," *NCP Guide* #1:50, 2nd. Ed., Nurseco, 1980.

The Diabetics Sports and Exercise Book, by J. Biermann and B. Toohey. J.B. Lippincott Co., Philadelphia, 1977.

"Travel Tips for the Peripatetic Diabetic," by Catherine Garofano. *Nursing 77*, August 1977:44–46.

"When a Pregnant Woman Is Diabetic." *American Journal of Nursing*, March 1979:448–458.

The Patient with Emphysema, Pulmonary

Definition: An irreversible condition in which there is dilatation of all the finer air passages, plus dilatation and coalesence of the alveoli resulting in loss of elasticity, trapping of air, and chronic hyperextension of the lungs.

LONG TERM GOAL: The patient will carry out activities of daily living within limitations and regimen imposed by the medical diagnosis, and will learn preventive measures designed to retard progress of the disease.

General Considerations:

— Pulmonary emphysema is one of three conditions collectively known as chronic, obstructive pulmonary disease (COPD); the other two are chronic bronchitis and asthma. Frequently, patients suffer from elements of all three.

— It usually **occurs** as the end result of chronic bronchial irritation and infection, which leads to edema, mucus production, bronchospasm, constriction of the finer airways, and loss of lung elasticity. It occurs most often in persons over 45 years of age who have a long history of cigarette smoking.

— There is no cure for the disease but its progress can be arrested in great part by maintenance of good, general health, avoidance of smoking, and control of air pollution.

— **Nursing responsibilities** include carrying out measures to resolve the acute conditions and teaching the patient/family/significant other preventive measures which will arrest progress of the disease and maintain optional pulmonary function.

Specific Considerations, Potential Patient Outcomes, and Nursing Actions:

1) Respiratory Dysfunction

The patient will maintain a patent airway; will breathe with as little effort as possible; will expectorate mucus:

— place pt. in an upright position, supporting back & arms (with pillow on over-bed table);

— check with Dr. re: giving O_2; the usual amt. is 1-2 liters/min., *no more* than 3 (otherwise, pt. may retain CO_2 which could lead to respiratory arrest); if O_2 given, administer it *continuously*, not intermittently;

— instruct pt. to use pursed-lip breathing during episodes of dypsnea;

— know that these pts. produce large amts. of thick sputum that is difficult to expectorate; suction PRN;

— provide adequate hydration (to liquefy secretions); check with Dr. re: fluid restrictions (related to existing cardiac or fluid problems); with no restrictions, ensure an intake of at least 2000cc's daily;

— provide humidification with warm steam or as Dr. orders, to aid expectoration;

— work with respiratory therapist re: scheduling of treatments & follow-up measures; with no respiratory therapist available, collaborate with Dr. re: postural drainage, IPPB & percussion/vibration to lower lobes;

— explain to pt. how the acute conditions (infection, respiratory failure/acidosis or whatever they are) impact upon his breathing & the expected results of treatment; be aware that acute SOB is a very frightening experience for the pt. & that giving information is an effective way to decrease fear & anxiety.

— observe for early signs of CO_2 narcosis (confusion, lethargy, deep sleep, changes in respiratory rate or depth, inability to help with own care) & report to Dr. at once; DC O_2.

2) Control of Infection

The patient will achieve resolution of acute episode; will be free of preventable infections:
— give antibiotics on time to maintain a constant level in blood;
— place pt. in a private room if possible, or at least away from any pt. with an infection;
— know that these pts. are especially susceptible to infections due to their chronic, debilitated condition;
— prevent staff & visitors with colds or other infections from going into pt.'s room;
— keep a large supply of tissues at bedside within easy reach of pt.;
— ensure that room is damp-dusted in an effort to cut down air pollution;
— check environmental controls: avoid draughts, chilling, extreme temperatures.

3) Energy Conservation

The patient will spread out energy demands over the day; the patient will avoid becoming extremely fatigued:
— know that these pts. have a limited amt. of energy, that energy is one of their most precious commodities, & that much of it is consumed with eating & talking;
— be aware that these pts. will have less energy in early am. due to accumulation of secretions during the night; postpone am. activities until they have expectorated the mucus;
— help pt. discover own point of fatigue, & to not go beyond that;
— ensure that pt. knows & carries out breathing exercises on a daily basis, & knows how to do pursed-lip breathing;
— keep pt.'s supplies close at hand so that s/he can reach them easily;
— schedule adequate rest periods between treatments, meals, tests, visitors, etc. to prevent pt. from becoming fatigued.

4) Patient Teaching Program

The patient will be able to do postural drainage, breathing exercises; will develop a plan to conserve energy:
— assess pt.'s ability to carry out postural drainage, percussion & vibration; collaborate with respiratory therapist to teach these procedures PRN;
— check pt.'s status re: breathing exercises; if pt. needs to strengthen muscles of expiration, suggest this:
   a) Do for 10-15 mins. TID: Patient in recumbent position, with one hand on abdomen and other on upper chest; inhale through nose, raising abdomen against hand; exhale while pursing lips, contracting the abdominal muscles, and moving abdomen inward; chest should not move. As patient can tolerate it, sand bags may be added to increase intra-abdominal pressure.

b) Do for 10 mins. TID: Take a full deep breath. Exhale slowly with pursed lips, blowing out a candle flame. but not extinguishing it. Flame should be 6" away; gradually increase 2" day to a distance of 36".
— as the acute condition resolves, ensure that pt. takes an active part in his care; allowing him to "just sit" & not participate may literally be deadly for him; his life depends upon learning to provide himself with an adequate pulmonary toilet:
— discuss with pt. his needs for rest, exercise, activity & help him adjust his energy resources accordingly:
— discuss the impact of air pollution, smoking, infections on his body; teach the action & possible side effects of his medications; teach signs of an impending problem or URI (chest tightness, change in color or amt. of sputum. chest pain. excessive fatigue); discuss the role of adequate nutrition & prevention of infection.

Discharge Planning and Teaching Objectives/Outcomes
1) (Patient/Family/Significant Other) Accepts diagnosis and recognizes that life can be useful, satisfying and worthwhile; knows that pulmonary function can be improved and maintained by adherence to prescribed regimen.
2) Verbalizes knowledge of the purpose and demonstrates satisfactorily postural drainage, aerosol therapy, breathing exercises, and room humidifiers.
3) States the actions and possible side effects of medication s/he is taking; has a supply of medicines to take home and knows where and when to obtain refills.
4) Identifies adequate knowledge of signs and symptoms of impending infection or other problems and knows to contact Dr./clinic at once.
5) Gives evidence of planning to maintain good health habits (adequate food and fluid intake, realistic level of rest and exercise, prevention of infection, avoidance of crowds, smoke-filled rooms, and air pollution.)

Recommended References
"Acute Respiratory Insufficiency," by Hannelore Sweetwood, RN, BS. *Nursing '77*, December 1977:24–31.
"Better Ways to Cope With C.O.P.D.," by Margaret F. Fuhr, RN, MSN and Alice M. Stein, RN, MA. *Nursing '76*, February 1976:28–38.
Fall-Winter Advice for Patients With Respiratory Problems. Respicare Service of Union Carbide Corp., 3 Westchester Plaza. Elmsford, NY 10523.
"Teaching Patients: General Suggestions," *NCP Guide* #1:49, 2nd Ed., Nurseco, 1980
"Teaching Patients: Specific Plan for Skills and Procedures," *NCP Guide* #1:50, 2nd Ed., Nurseco, 1980.

The Patient with a Hemorrhoidectomy

Definition: Hemorrhoidectomy is a surgical ligation and excision of the dilated blood vessels in the anal region, external to the sphincter and, if needed, submucosal vessels above the internal sphincter.

LONG TERM GOAL: The patient will recover from a hemorrhoidectomy free of complications; the patient will return to usual roles in home/job/community after a normal short convalescence.

General Considerations:
— **Medical treatment** for small hemorrhoids that are mild and uncomplicated consists of a low roughage diet, increased exercise for those with sedentary lifestyles, sitz baths for relief of pain and itching, anesthetic ointments, stool softeners and lubricant suppositories.
— Fear of surgery and pain cause many persons to refuse surgery for as long as possible, even after several episodes of severe pain, bleeding, prolapse and near strangulation. Nurses can help people to reduce their anxiety and to accept an operation when it is recommended.
— **Preop nursing care responsibilities** include operative and anesthetic consents, a perianal prep, tap water enemas until clear, liquid low residue diet, pre-anesthetic medications, voiding or foley catheter placement and oft needed reassurance and explanations.

Specific Postop Considerations, Potential Patient Outcomes and Nursing Actions:

1) Rest and Comfort

The patient will experience prompt, effective relief of pain as needed; the patient will experience reduced tension, embarrassment, aggression and other nonproductive behaviors associated with severe anal discomfort:
— give narcotics & sedatives as frequently as ordered; don't wait for pt. requests which may be delayed for one reason or another;
— keep fresh ice packs over anal dressing until packing is removed; then astringent, tepid, moist compresses may be ordered;
— anesthetic/antibiotic ointments may be ordered, although excessive use may delay wound healing;
— position pt. on abdomen or side with pillow supports;
— change dressings, T-binders, bedding to keep area clean, dry, comfortable;
— have pt. take 15-20 min. warm sitz baths QID & PRN; have a foam ring or towel in tub for sitting comfort; observe for dizziness, oversedation or weakness & do not leave pt. alone;
— show sympathetic, sensitive, yet tactful concern; avoid embarrassing remarks or questionable humor.

2) Prevention of Complications	The patient will have bleeding and infection prevented or promptly controlled:

2) Prevention of Complications — The patient will have bleeding and infection prevented or promptly controlled:
— monitor & record TPR and B/P noting quality & changes;
— note restlessness, anxiety, weakness or other behavior change;
— observe for continuing, bright red bleeding & passage of clots; report this to doctor, put pt. to bed, apply ice bag over an absorbent pressure dressing & watch closely.

3) Nutrition — The patient will resume a regular diet as tolerated after initially taking a liquid to soft low residue diet:
— give liquid to soft low residue diet to postpone first defecation until some healing has taken place & there is less chance of bleeding or infection;
— after recording the first bowel movement, a regular diet is given.

4) Voiding — The patient will resume normal urinary output without bladder distention:
— urge & record oral fluids, especially tea & coffee if permitted;
— palpate supra-pubic region for distention or ascertain that catheter (if placed) is unkinked & continually patent;
— measure each voided amt. separately to assess retention;
— help male pts. stand to void; help females into sitting position on bedside commode; rinse perineum & change anal dressing after voiding;
— try sitz baths (or Urecholine type injections if ordered) to stimulate voiding & avoid catheterization except as a last resort.

5) Defecation — The patient will achieve satisfactory bowel movements with as little strain and pain as possible:
— administer laxatives & low retention enema when ordered;
— have pt. take a sitz bath prior to defecation attempt in order to relax & to facilitate removal of cellulose gauze spool used for hemostasis;
— administer narcotic injection for pain relief at least 20-30 min. prior to elimination effort;
— help pt. to bathroom, provide privacy, but remain close by in case of dizziness or other need;
— after defecation, have pt. rest for a few minutes, then take a short sitz bath to cleanse peri-anal region & to promote healing & comfort.

Discharge Planning and Teaching Objectives/Outcomes

1) (Patient/Family/Significant Other) Has written appointment, date and time for follow-up visit to surgeon.
2) Has obtained (or knows how to get) a foam ring or cushion for sitting comfort.
3) States s/he knows about diet, laxatives, pain medications, sitz baths, safety precautions, need for exercise and expectations for being permitted to drive a car, sit for long periods, return to work, etc.

The Patient with Hepatitis

Definition: Hepatitis is an inflammation and injury of the liver caused by chemical substances (toxic hepatitis), different viruses or other organisms, e.g. gonococcus, streptococcus (viral hepatitis).

LONG TERM GOAL: The patient will accept illness and recover to the point that s/he is willing and able to complete convalescence at home with medical guidance; the patient will return to normal roles in home/job/community.

General Considerations:
— **Signs and Symptoms:** dark urine, clay-colored stools, yellow sclera, jaundice, N&V, anorexia, fatigue, malaise, myalgia, headache, fever; may also have cough, pharyngitis, photophobia; rash, hives, edema and pruritis also possible.
— Viral hepatitis is most commonly of two types: serum hepatitis (type B) or infectious hepatitis (type A). **Both** may be transmitted orally (food, water, fingers contaminated by urine, feces, saliva, semen) or parenterally (blood or blood product-contaminated syringes, needles, dental & surgical instruments, ear piercing tools, etc.) A new Type C Hepatitis has been found in patients who have had multiple transfusions.
— **Incubation period:** 2-4 mos. for SH and 2-8 wks. for IH; exceptions have been recorded.
— **Treatment** to heal and regenerate the liver depends upon adequate rest (often in bed, 2 weeks to 2 months) and a balanced, nutritious, high carbohydrate-low fat diet. Regularly repeated liver function blood studies (SGOT, SGPT, alkaline phosphatase, serum bilirubin, iceterus index, pro time) indicate the effectiveness of treatment and progress of recovery (4-24 weeks).
— **Nursing responsibilities** include health teaching, isolation precautions and procedures designed to minimize outbreaks (e.g. careful handling of bodily secretions, blood and blood products, needles and syringes; no eating policies in hemodialysis, oncology, hematology or blood-donor units; proper housekeeping practices and thorough hand washing habits before and after patient care).

Specific Considerations, Potential Patient Outcomes, and Nursing Actions:
1) Rest and Comfort

The patient's liver cells will heal and regenerate with minimal residual liver damage:
— bed rest for one or more weeks with use of private bath & toilet facilities is common, if pt. was previously healthy;
— passive & active range-of-motion exercises should be taught & done twice daily; refer to NCPG #1:47;
— provide stress-reducing activities that will encourage rest & relaxation; arrange for sensory stimulation (TV, radio, books, clock, calendar, pictures, hobbies, etc.) & social contacts (visits by friends, family & available staff);
— query pt. re: medications being taken; those which are metabolized in the liver (birth control pills, Dilantin, sedatives, tranquilizers, others) are to be avoided during the acute illness period;
— provide regular skin care, using baths & lotions for dry, itching skin; use decubitus & pressure prevention measures.

2) Nutrition

The patient maintains an optimum fluid, electrolyte, nutritional balance refraining from foods and liquids harmful to the liver:
— administer parenteral fluids with vitamin & mineral supplements as prescribed during the acute phase, especially when the

pt. is anorexic, or has nausea & vomiting;
— when tolerated, serve Hi Pro-Hi CHO-Lo Fat diet in six, small feedings daily; arrange for someone to be present so pt. does not have to eat alone; consult dietician for cultural preferences or special needs;
— hard candy to increase carbohydrate level is no longer advised because it further depresses the appetite for nutritious foods; instead, fresh or canned fruits & juices are provided & encouraged;
— alcohol must be avoided for 4-6 mos. to prevent relapse or prolong convalescence; peanuts, chocolate, ice cream and other fatty foods & snacks are to be avoided as well.

3) Isolation Precautions   The spread of the hepatitis virus will be contained and cross-contamination will be prevented:
— wear gowns, but caps & masks are usually not necessary; gloves are recommended for handling all body secretions;
— tissues, toothbrushes, bed linens, other patient care items require special handling according to hospital procedure;
— carefully dispose of all disposable needles, syringes, IV equipment, paper food service items;
— teach pt. & family necessary precautions, indicating which will be continued after the pt. goes home; kissing is not permitted; the pt. must not prepare or handle food for others; a private bathroom should be provided or care taken to keep the basin and toilet scrupulously clean;
— hand washing is a must for staff, visitors & pt.; a mask should be worn by the pt. if s/he is prone to coughing, sneezing;
— reassure pt. that precautions are temporary; pt. should not be rejected, left alone for long periods or neglected.

4) Prevention of Complications   The patient will be free of preventable complications or have them promptly recognized and managed:
— observe & record changes in pt.'s physical or mental status; note signs of disorientation, irritability, depression; look for ascites, edema, asterixis (metabolic tremor);
— note new bruises or petechiae; observe bleeding from needle sites;
— record color of urine & stools, observing for presence of bleeding, & signs of shock that come with blood loss.

Discharge Planning and Teaching Objectives/Outcomes

1) (Patient/Family/Significant Other) Understands status of own hepatitis and expresses willingness to adhere to treatment.
2) Has a written list of foods permitted and disallowed on diet; can state a typical day's menu; indicates an appreciation of need to eat at least every three hours to spare liver from unnecessary metabolic work.
3) Has been assisted to complete job disability insurance forms and to make home care arrangements according to need. Knows s/he must not return to any strenuous work or fatiguing activities until doctor has given permission.

Recommended References
"Range of Motion Exercises," *NCP Guide* #1:47, 2nd Ed., Nurseco, 1980.
"Viral Hepatitis," by Karen Baranowski, Harry Green II, and J. Thomas Lamont. *Nursing 76*, May 1976:31–38.

The Patient with Hypertension

Definition: Hypertension, according to the American Heart Association, is simply an unstable or persistent elevation of blood pressure above the normal range.

LONG TERM GOAL: The patient will reach an optimum level of functioning within a therapeutic program and a modified lifestyle necessary to control his blood pressure throughout his life.

General Considerations:

— Persons with a consistent **systolic BP reading equal to or greater than 160 mm. Hg. and a diastolic reading greater than 90 mm. Hg.,** generally are considered to be hypertensive and in need of medical evaluation.

— **Incidence:** Estimated at one adult in six in US; more prevalent in women, in black people, often those between 30 & 50 years of age, and in obese persons. Most hypertensives are undiagnosed because of a lack of symptoms ("the hidden disease"); of those who are known, most have "primary" or "essential" type.

— **Causes & Types:** Kidney disease, an adrenal tumor, toxemia of pregnancy and birth control pills are sometimes causes of high blood pressure. In the absence of a known cause, hypertension is typed *essential* or *primary*. It may also be classified as *benign* (slow onset, minimal symptoms) or *malignant* (degenerated and occluded peripheral blood vessels).

— **Treatment aims:** To reduce arterial pressure, to arrest atherosclerosis and to curtail progressive arteriolar disease. To maintain the blood pressure within safe levels, a patient must faithfully adhere to a program of diet, drugs, balanced rest/relaxation/exercise/work schedule and periodic medical check-ups.

— **Low compliance** is a major (& common, 3 out of 4) problem among hypertensives. Reasons given by patients for discontinuing treatment regimen include: felt well, couldn't afford medications, had disagreeable side effects from prescribed drugs, feared dependency on drugs, felt embarrassed or guilty about need to take medicine daily even when symptom-free, received poor or inadequate instruction from medical personnel, took conflicting advice of friends, and/or became discouraged or dissatisfied with continuing treatment, long waits and seeing different doctors during clinic visits, and depersonalization attitude of professional staff.

— **Nursing responsibilities:** Case-finding efforts to detect the unknown, untreated hypertensive; assessment of patient & family for planning, implementing and evaluating a simple, satisfying and successful treatment regimen; and effective education to ensure life-long compliance. Close cooperation between nursing colleagues in the out-patient and in-patient settings (including community health staff) is important to obtain cooperation of patient and a consistent, congruent approach to patient/family.

— The **patient must "own" his disease**, assume responsibility for own health, but must be made to feel that someone cares whether s/he does or not. Support should come from loving family members, concerned significant others and empathetic health care providers. If s/he is to avoid repeated hospitalizations and a worsening illness (serious complications are myocardial infarction, congestive heart failure, stroke and progressive renal failure), s/he must **accept** lifelong hypertensive condition requiring medication to control it even when s/he doesn't feel bad.

Specific Considerations, Potential Patient Outcomes, and Nursing Actions:

1) Nutrition   The patient will accept and adhere to a low sodium, weight control diet to eliminate overweight, to prevent edema, to reduce the work load of the heart and to lower the blood pressure to satisfactory levels:

— assess pt. attitudes toward food, cooking, seasonings & meal times, so as to gauge motivation to learn & to plan more effective teaching;
— estimate the probable effect that altered food preparation will have on family; learn the family's attitude, beliefs about the pt.'s need for special diet & the degree of willingness to cooperate;
— teach pt./family that sodium restriction will reduce blood volume, thereby lessening the work of the heart;
— confer with dietician re: pt.'s likes & dislikes, cultural preferences, special needs, in order to plan an acceptable diet while in the hospital & to teach effectively about the diet recommended after discharge;
— help the pt. to understand & accept a low sodium weight control diet;
— record daily weight & I & O; note foods left on tray & discuss reason;
— teach pt. what food seasonings do not contain sodium & what salt substitutes are permissible & safe to use; teach pt. to check food labels carefully for sodium compounds;
— teach pt. that caffeine is a vasoconstrictor which increases heart's work & that coffee, tea, cola drinks & chocolate have caffeine;
— refer to NCPG #3:44, "Low Sodium Diets";
— give pt./family written dietary instructions to read & keep.

2) Rest and   The patient will experience reduced physical and emotional tension; the patient's circulation and muscle tone will be improved;
   Exercise   the patient will explore new ways of coping more effectively with stress:

— recommend & provide for daily walks, up to 30 min. depending on physical status & activity tolerance;
— encourage the pt. to decide to participate more actively in some sport (golf, tennis, bowling, ball games, bicycling, etc.) when s/he is discharged;
— teach progressive muscle relaxation exercises & relaxed breathing techniques (such as natural childbirth type or hatha yoga type); see recommended references below;
— discuss with pt. the need for & value of daily quiet periods alone with self & for occasional long weekends in some leisure activity;
— investigate the possibility of biofeedback therapy to help pt. develop self control of muscular & nervous tension;

— consult with occupational & recreational therapy for appropriate relaxation suggestions (e.g. needlepointing, painting, learning to play a musical instrument, etc.);

— know that sedatives & tranquilizers are not effective in lowering BP & generally are not recommended for taking on a regular basis.

3) Drug Therapy The patient achieves a stable BP within physician-determined parameters; the patient is able to cope adaptively with drug's side effects, stating s/he realizes that the side effects are less dangerous than the effects of not taking the antihypertensive drug:

— know the expected & desired action of each drug given as well as the untoward effects to be observed & recorded; teach this to pt. & family; diuretics, sympathetic nervous system inhibitors and/or smooth muscle vasodilators may be given, but an attempt will be made to achieve sufficient reduction of BP with the lowest possible dosage of the fewest number of drugs, so it is important for the nurse to observe carefully & record accurately the pt.'s response to drug(s);

— question how the pt. feels & include the family's observations; side effects may include dry mouth, fatigue, diarrhea, depression, GI disturbances, drowsiness & others;

— observe for signs of potassium loss (calf or leg cramps, weakness, fatigue, mental confusion, apathy); check serum potassium level; for hypokalemia, pt. can eat foods high in potassium (raisins, prunes, orange juice, bananas, fish, leafy green veg.), can substitute KCL table salt for Na Cl, & doctor may order a potassium supplement; refer to NCPG #2:48, "Potassium Imbalance";

— if pt. is on a potassium-conserving diuretic, observe for signs of hyponatremia (lowered blood sodium: thirst, diminished sweating, fever, weakness, confusion) & hyperkalemia (weakness, numbness & tingling in extremities, slower pulse than normal, listlessness); pt. should **not** use a potassium-containing salt substitute, in this case;

— force fluids; dehydration from fever or hot weather enhances potency of hypotensive drugs;

— monitor & record TPR & BP when ordered & at other times to provide a guide or indication of drug effectiveness; note the pt.'s position (sitting, standing, lying down) & other pertinent variables (exercise, emotional reaction); keep the pt. informed of BP & let him assist in record keeping, so that s/he will feel informed & responsible for his own progress;

— watch for signs of orthostatic (postural) hypotension (dizziness, light-headedness); have pt. sit or squat down at first sign of weakness to prevent serious injuries from falls; teach pt. to assume a sitting position (after lying down) *slowly*, then a standing position while holding onto something, then a pause, before starting to walk;

— explore with pt./family any concerns or misconceptions s/he may have about taking medication daily for most of life; know that common feelings include embarrassment, guilt, fear of dependency, distrust of dosage amounts, disbelief & denial of need to take medications after s/he feels better, dismay over continuing cost of drugs; distress over unpleasant side effects & fear of sexual dysfunction which can occur as a side effect of some drugs; tell pt. that alternate drugs & dosages can be tried if side effects are intolerable, but that s/he must take some hypotensive drug(s) to keep BP under control;

— teach pt. to avoid over-the-counter cold remedies (which often contain vasoconstrictors) & aspirin compounds (which may contain caffeine) because these will interfere with their antihypertensive therapy;

— counsel & support pt. efforts to reduce or stop smoking; explain that nicotine is a vasoconstrictor & therefore increases the heart's work load; do not permit visitors to smoke in front of pt. & arrange for nonsmokers as pt. roommates;

— with the pt. & family, establish a medication routine that reduces the chance of error & forgetting; devise a simple schedule around the pt.'s work & sleep habits.

4) Psychosocial Adjustment

The patient accepts hypertension as a lifelong condition requiring continuing treatment; the patient expresses a firm commitment to actively participate in treatment program; the patient expresses fears, needs, and concerns to a receptive, empathetic professional person:

— know that common fears & problems of hypertensives include: denial (of need to know about hypertension, of symptoms, of need to take medications when feeling good), excessive anxiety & tension, reluctance to be physically active, fear of missing too much work or failing to get a promotion because of repeated doctor appointments, misconceptions about hypertension disease, treatment & control; encourage pt./family to express these concerns; ask them what this condition will mean to pt. in terms of how s/he sees himself & lifestyle;

— assess pt.'s orientation to health, its value, pt.'s belief in prevention or only in cure; find out what pt. knows & determine what s/he needs & wants to know; help pt. identify own risk factors & the lifestyle changes s/he is willing to make to obtain control of condition;

— find out the possible obstacles to pt. keeping appointments, taking prescribed medications, adhering to diet, coping with stress, stopping smoking, exercising daily, & continuing to monitor own BP;

— answer questions, correct errors & gaps in knowledge, provide necessary information; evaluate & record what has been learned & determine what reinforcement & reminders will be needed;

— obtain a written or verbal commitment to comply with treatment regimen which pt. has had an opportunity to help plan & to express feelings & reactions concerning it; support & encourage pt.'s positive attitude & intentions to cooperate.

Discharge Planning and Teaching Objectives/Outcomes

1) (Patient/Family/Significant Other) Can explain own specific pathology, its ramifications, what contributes to his disease process and the consequences of non-treatment.

2) Demonstrates an understanding of the what, why and when of total antihypertensive treatment program for own condition. Expresses willingness to assume responsibility for control of own BP and gives a commitment to follow treatment regimen faithfully.

3) Has received, read and understands written dietary instructions; can plan a typical day's menu and tell what is permitted or disallowed on the diet.

4) For each drug to be taken, know its purpose, schedule of dosage and untoward side effects to be observed and reported to doctor. Can express knowledge that his medications will help to keep his blood pressure down, only if s/he takes them continually on a regular basis, exactly as ordered, even after s/he feels completely well again.

5) Has received at least one descriptive pamphlet on hypertension, with doctor's approval, and has at least one community health resource person's name and number for getting further help and information (in addition to his doctor).

6) Can take own blood pressure accurately and knows when to notify doctor of results. (Get doctor's approval for teaching patient this technique.)

7) Has a follow-up appointment and promises (or contracts) to keep it.

Recommended References

"Breathing Techniques That Help Reduce Hypertension," by Sharon Dowdall. *RN*, October 1977:73–76.

"Diets: Low Sodium." *NCP Guide #3:44*, Nurseco, 1977.

"Guidelines for Educating Nurses in High Blood Pressure Control." High Blood Pressure Information Center, 120/80, National Institutes of Health, Bethesda, MD 20014.

"Helping The Hypertensive Patient Control Sodium Intake," by Martha Hill. *American Journal of Nursing*, May 1979:906–909.

"Helping Your Hypertensive Patients Live Longer," by Rosemary Maloney. *Nursing 78*, October 1978:26–34.

High Blood Pressure (Hypertension) and *Your Blood Pressure* (leaflets), American Heart Assn., 7320 Greenville Ave., Dallas, TX 75231.

"Potassium Imbalance." *NCP Guide #2:48*, 2nd. Ed., Nurseco, 1980.

"Promoting Patient Adherence," by Sue Foster and Deborah Kousch. *American Journal of Nursing*, May 1978:829–832.

"Protocol for Teaching Hypertensive Patients," by Ellen Mitchell. *American Journal of Nursing*, May 1977:808,809.

"Treating and Counseling the Hypertensive Patient," by Graham Ward et al. *American Journal of Nursing*, May 1978:824–828.

Understanding High Blood Pressure, Searle and Co., PO Box 5110, Chicago, IL 60680.

The Patient with a Hysterectomy

Definition: Hysterectomy is removal of the uterus: total (including tubes and ovaries) or sub-total (only the uterus), also known as a partial hysterectomy.

LONG TERM GOAL: The patient will return to her optimum level of health and resume usual roles in home, family, community after a normal, short convalescence following safe, successful removal of uterus; the patient will accept and cope effectively with her altered body image and loss.

General Considerations:
— Removal of the uterus may be done by abdominal or vaginal routes, depending on surgical diagnosis. Surgery may include A&P repair (anterior and posterior colporraphy—vaginal suture) for cystocele and rectocele (prolapses of bladder and rectum). Nursing care will vary accordingly, but principles re: restoration of normal function, prevention of complications, psycho-social adjustment remain essentially the same.

— **Preoperative nursing responsibility** is that for general abdominal surgery with the addition of a complete perineal prep and a cleansing douche, as ordered. Refer to NCPG #2:44, "General Preoperative Nursing Care." In addition, provide the patient with the information and reassurance she wants or needs re: hospitalization (usually a week or less), the operation, the expected post-operative course and convalescence. Nurses should be aware of what this operation means to patient so as to avoid inadvertent casualness or oversolicitude. Normal concerns include those of dying, of cancer, of disfigurement, of loss of femininity and sexuality, of pain, of loss of childbearing ability, of ability to cope or control destiny and of weight gain or other menopausal changes. The reactions and attitudes of husband, family and friends will affect the perceptions and the post-operative adjustment of the patient, as well as the length of convalescence.

— **Postoperative nursing responsibility** is that for general abdominal surgery (and is less complex for vaginal approach). Refer to NCPGs #2:41, 42, 43, "General Postoperative Nursing Care, Part A, Part B, & Part C." In addition, see NCPG #1:31, "Responses to Loss: the Grief and Mourning Process," and NCPG #2:29, "The Patient Experiencing a Body Image Disturbance." Most women under 40 can resume normal activities in a month and will feel quite like themselves or better in about two months. Older women in less ideal physical condition will need longer to regain strength and vitality.

Specific Considerations, Potential Patient Outcomes, and Nursing Actions:

1) General
   Abdominal
   Surgery
   Post-Op
   Measures

The patient will resume normal cardio-pulmonary function and fluid and electrolyte balance; the patient will be free of preventable complications:
— turn, cough, deep breathe & turn pt. Q2H;
— monitor & record TPR & BP according to standard postop routine until stable;
— monitor & record parenteral fluids; record I & O;
— administer antibiotics, vitamins & minerals, sedatives & analgesics as ordered; observe for untoward reactions;
— give food & fluids as tolerated when parenteral fluids are dc'ed & peristalsis returns;
— keep in low Fowler's or flat position to prevent increased intra-abdominal pressure; apply abdominal binder for additional support & comfort;
— give passive & active leg exercises at least Q4H; use elastic bandages for legs from ankle to groin & re-wrap Q8H; do not flex thighs sharply or place pt. in a high Fowler's position; leg dangling & progressive ambulation should be done as soon as surgeon permits.

2) Elimination

The patient will maintain adequate output and normal elimination will be restored after sutured area has begun sufficient healing:
— check indwelling catheter for patency & avoid dependent loops hanging below bed level;
— prevent bladder infection by sterile handling of tubes when disconnecting; use antibiotic ointment around meatus; obtain urine specimens from catheter with syringe & needle, using sterile technique;
— refer to NCPG #2:39, "Catheters: Indwelling Urinary";
— after catheter removal, check voiding Q4H; measure amt. voided; notify doctor if voiding frequent, small amts. or if unable to void in 6 hrs. if intake has been adequate; observe for signs of bladder infection;
— if rectocele has been repaired, a liquid low residue diet may be ordered to delay first defecation; then mineral oil laxatives and oil retention enemas are given to lubricate & ease movement without strain.

3) Perineal Care
   (for A-P Repair)
   & Dressings

The patient will heal with a minimum of discomfort and without infection:
— cleanse perineum with prescribed sterile solution twice daily & after each elimination; use heat lamp to help dry area & to promote healing;
— give sitz baths after sutures are removed for cleansing & comfort;
— for vaginal hysterectomy, encourage pts. to shower when able;
— check perineal pads to describe color, amt. & odor of drainage;
— for abdominal hysterectomy, reinforce dressing PRN; note amt. bleeding & report changes in pt. status.

4) Psychosocial
   Adjustment

The patient will adapt effectively to trauma of surgery, to her loss of uterus and altered body image; the patient will express growing confidence in ability to cope:

— teach & convince pt. that depression, weepiness, worry, helplessness & other seemingly unreasonable behavior are normal & expected; assure her that her ability to cope & remain in control will return in due course;

— help family & friends understand her need for repeated assurances of their love, concern & availability; encourage them to support her attractiveness & self-esteem; explore their cultural attitudes re: the female role in order to learn its probable effect on pt.'s perceptions:

— provide regular opportunities for talking, asking questions, expressing feelings & planning for future;

— re: intercourse, it is often helpful to say, "If you enjoyed it before, you will enjoy it afterwards," and vice versa; ending fears of pregnancy and relieving symptoms often improve intercourse but do not raise false hopes;

— provide copy of *After Hysterectomy, What?* (see ref.).

Discharge Planning and Teaching Objectives/Outcomes

1) (Patient/Family/Significant Other) Knows what surgery has been done and what changes in herself to expect (menopausal symptoms, effects of hormonal therapy, weakness, fatigue, irritability & crying are customary) during convalescence.

2) Knows to avoid sexual intercourse, heavy lifting, vacuuming, pushing a full grocery cart, driving or prolonged sitting in a car, active sports or other "jarring" activities until doctor's approval (usually 4 to 8 weeks).

3) Knows that spotting and changing perineal pad twice daily is normal, but to report frank bleeding, increasing amounts of discharge or malodorous discharge promptly to doctor.

4) Understands and accepts responsibility for convalescence which may include: sitz baths, laxatives and medication for discomfort and rest, slow and moderate exercise with intermittent rest periods, a balanced diet and, for some, possible use of a girdle and support stockings. Knows that for some women, at least 9 weeks to three months may be required to "feel like themselves" again, depending on a variety of influencing factors (physical condition, mental attitude, increased age, attitude of family and friends, etc.).

Recommended References

After Hysterectomy, What? by Lindsay R. Curtis. ℅ Mallicote Printing, 509 Shelby St., Bristol, Tenn.

"Catheters: Indwelling, Urethral." NCP Guide #2:39, 2nd Ed., Nurseco, 1980.

"Easier Convalescence from Hysterectomy," by Margaret Williams. *American Journal of Nursing*, March 1978:438–440.

"General Postoperative Nursing Care, Part A, Part B, Part C." *NCP Guides* #2:41, 42, 43, 2nd Ed., Nurseco, 1980.

"General Preoperative Nursing Care," *NCP Guide* #2:44, 2nd Ed., Nurseco, 1980.

"Responses to Loss: the Grief and Mourning Process," *NCP Guide* #1:31, 2nd Ed., Nurseco, 1980.

"The Patient Experiencing a Body Image Disturbance," *NCP Guide* #2:29, 2nd Ed., Nurseco, 1980.

The Patient with an Ileostomy

Definition: Ileostomy is a surgically constructed bowel outlet on the abdomen, using the ileum.

LONG TERM GOAL: The patient will recover from a successful ileostomy without preventable complications, returning to optimum health and usual roles in home, job, community after a normal convalescence; the patient will accept and cope realistically and adaptively to an altered body image and loss of normal elimination function.

General Considerations:

— **Incidence:** There are approximately 1,500,000 ostomates in North America with nearly 100,000 new ostomy surgeries per year. Diseases which commonly necessitate ileostomy are chronic, advanced ulcerative colitis, familial polyposis, and Crohn's Disease (granulomatous colitis).

— **Ileostomy involves** the removal of the entire colon. The end of the ileum is brought out to the abdomen, forming a stoma. Fecal discharge is continuous or intermittent, but cannot be completely regulated and a collection bag is worn cemented to the skin. Some surgeons in a few large medical centers are now creating an internal pouch which retains ileal contents until the patient is ready to empty it at his convenience. The procedure, called a "continent" ileostomy, is still somewhat experimental since 1971, and is not recommended for obese patients or patients with regional ileitis or cancer.

— A proctectomy (removal of rectum) is usually also done. If not, the patient will have periodic mucus discharge from rectum and should be told this.

— **Nursing responsibilities** include (1) physical preoperative preparation of the patient with the usual measures for general abdominal surgery, i.e. operative and anesthesia consents, skin prep, nasogastric intubation, restriction of food and fluids, cleansing enemas, antibacterial medications and pre-anesthetic sedation. Refer to Nursing Care Planning Guide #2:44, "General Preoperative Nursing Care." (2) Provision for intellectual acceptance and emotional assimilation, preoperatively, by one or more of the following measures: have an enterostomal therapist, a mental health clinician or consultant, a qualified nurse or a selected ileostomate talk with patient, giving him an opportunity to ask questions, express concerns, seek reassurance, correct misconceptions and learn about the postoperative regimen. Normal fears are those of dying, of cancer, of pain, of disfigurement, of loss of sexuality, of inability to control body and what happens and of changed body image and self-concept. Actually sickness and disability have so changed the patient's lifestyle that an ileostomy is often a welcome release and afterward, most patients feel better than they have for years.

Specific Considerations, Potential Patient Outcomes, and Nursing Actions:

1) General
Abdominal
Surgery
Postop
Measures

The patient maintains adequate cardio-pulmonary, musculoskeletal and renal body functions; the patient is free of preventable complications of hemorrhage, infection, pneumonia and stomal damage; the patient is carefully monitored and free of complications of fluid loss, sodium and potassium deficit; the patient maintains adequate fluid and electrolyte balance:

— refer to NCPGs #2:41, 42, 43, "General Postoperative Nursing Care, Part A, Part B, Part C";
— monitor & record vital signs, CVP readings as ordered;
— monitor administration of parenteral fluids, electrolytes & vitamin supplements; refer to NCPG #2:46, "Intravenous Therapy: General Principles," NCPGs #3:48 & #3:49, "Fluids & Electrolytes, Part A & Part B";
— record I&O accurately; check urine output QH, recording specific gravity; watch closely for oliguria (reduced urine output);
— know that these pts. are especially vulnerable to fluid loss & electrolyte imbalance; watch for signs of sodium deficit (abdominal cramps, hypotension, rapid & thready pulse, apathy) & potassium deficit (weakness, paresthesias, faint irregular pulse, soft flabby muscles); refer to serum electrolyte reports & report promptly imbalances; see NCPG #2:48;
— turn, cough, & deep breathe pt. Q2H; have pt. exercise legs with each position change;
— keep nasogastric tube functioning & patent until peristalsis returns & tube is removed; record color & amt. drainage; provide oral hygiene Q2H;
— administer analgesics, sedatives, antibiotics as ordered.

2) Stomal Care

The patient will have adequate ileal drainage without blockage, leakage, skin irritation or odors; the patient will be able to care for own ileostomy.

— consult nearest local Enterostomal Therapist for information & help with pt.;
— observe & record color, amt. and consistency of ileostomy drainage; explain to pt. why drainage is watery & appliance needs frequent emptying to prevent pulling on the skin; empty when only 1/3 full;
— see NCPG #1:43, ". . . Changing a Temporary or Permanent Appliance"; note promptly & change a loosening or leaking appliance; prevent skin irritation with applications of plain tincture of benzoin & karaya gum rings or mixture;
— observe for peristomal monilia infection which is very common, especially in pts. on systemic antibiotics; look for erythematous center with a border of red papules; itching may be present; confirm with a culture; apply Mycostatin (R) Powder each time appliance is changed;
— observe & report stomal retraction or protrusion, peristomal skin irritation & infection; explain to pt. that stoma will continue to shrink in size for approx. 8 weeks as healing occurs & initial swelling subsides; tell pt. that some change in size & shape will also gradually occur over the first year; stress that because of this, it is necessary to measure stoma *each* time appliance is changed in order to fit the skin protective wafers & appliance *snugly* around stoma to prevent any leakage-caused skin excoriation;
— prevent & control humiliating odors by frequent emptying & rinsing of collection bag, by using deodorizing preparations

inside bag, by airing room after emptying bag, by using a room deodorant, & by having pt. take orally bismuth subgallate, N.F. for internal control of odor;

— encourage & provide means for pt. to assist & gradually assume care of own ileostomy as soon as s/he is physically & emotionally able; see NCPG #1:49, "Teaching Patients: General Suggestions," and NCPG #1:50, "Teaching Patients: Specific Plan for Skills & Procedures."

3) Nutrition   The patient will resume special diet as tolerated:

— gradually resume liquid, then soft, then regular consistency bland, low residue foods when nasogastric tube is removed; note pt. tolerance;

— introduce small amounts of each new food, noting intestinal reactions; teach pt. to do this at home;

— ask pt. to chew food completely, eating slowly to avoid blockage of ileum;

— know that severe gas pains are common; have pt. chew food with mouth closed, refrain from talking while eating, & avoid use of a straw for drinking liquids;

— teach pt. to avoid gas-forming foods such as beans, sauerkraut, cauliflower, cucumbers, onions, cabbage & carbonated drinks.

4) Psychosocial   The patient will adapt realistically to an altered body image and self-concept; the patient will cope effectively with the loss of
   Adjustment   normal body elimination, accepting ileostomy and caring for it with confidence; the family expresses understanding and acceptance of patient's altered condition and provides emotional support to patient:

— be sensitive to behavioral cues: depression, silence, apathy, refusal to cooperate may indicate feelings of anger, grief, loss of self-esteem due to the shocking physical reality of the operation; refer to NCPG #1:31, "Responses to Loss: the Grief and Mourning Process";

— see NCP Guides on specific behaviors (#'s1:20-33); discuss pt.'s responses with pt./family & nursing staff & work together toward understanding & realistic plans of care; write approaches in care plan;

— arrange to have a successfully rehabilitated ostomate visit pt.;

— encourage pt. to touch stoma; refer to NCPG #2:29, "The Patient Experiencing a Body Image Disturbance"; help pt. to express feelings & to face the reality of the surgical experience; include the spouse or significant other in the pt.'s life so that discussions can be more beneficial: identify their concerns & correct misconceptions; recognize intimacy as a valued need & help them to discuss this openly, yet with sensitivity & understanding;

— provide pt./family/significant other with informational booklets from the United Ostomy Assn.; see recommended references.

Discharge Planning and Teaching Objectives/Outcomes

1) (Patient/Family/Significant Other) States s/he knows basic facts re: diet, exercise, restriction of heavy lifting, medications (dosage, effects, untoward effects to be reported) returning to former job and activities.
2) Can describe the type of surgery and kind of stoma s/he has; demonstrates correct, safe confident care of ileostomy and appliance change.
3) Knows to report promptly to physician complications, abdominal cramps, vomiting, diarrhea, cessation of ileostomy drainage, pain, fever or other illness.
4) Has an identification card for wallet listing medications, routine of ileostomy care, the name and phone number of physician, and the next of kin to be notified in case of accident.
5) Has at least two weeks' ileostomy supplies and the name and address of local supplier for additional needs.
6) Has been evaluated for assistance (financial, vocational, social service disability, homemaker and home health care) and has received appropriate referrals.
7) Has the name and phone number of nearest local enterostomal theapist and/or community health nurse.
8) Knows how to handle *minor* episodes of constipation, diarrhea, and peristomal skin irritation.
9) Has received literature and information appropriate to needs and concerns; knows how to contact local ostomy association for further support services.
10) Has received the address of The United Ostomy Assn., Inc., 2001 Beverly Blvd., Los Angeles, CA 90057.

Recommended References
"Basic Principles for Changing a Temporary or Permanent Appliance," *NCP Guide* #1:43, 2nd Ed., Nurseco, 1980.
"Fluids & Electrolytes, Part A: Fluids, Part B: Electrolytes," *NCP Guides* #3:48 & 3:49, Nurseco, 1977.
"General Postoperative Nursing Care, Part A, Part B, Part C," *NCP Guides* #2:41, 2:42, 2:43, 2nd Ed., Nurseco, 1980.
"General Preoperative Nursing Care," *NCP Guide* #2:44, 2nd Ed., Nurseco, 1980.
"Helping the Ileostomy Patient to Help Himself," by Jacqueline Lamanske. *Nursing 77*, January 1977:34–39.
"If the Ileostomy Is Continent, the Benefits Are Obvious," by Charlotte Isler. *RN*, April 1977:39–45.
"Intravenous Therapy: General Principles," *NCP Guide* #2:46, 2nd Ed., Nurseco, 1980.
"PostOperative Education For the Ileostomate," by Debra Broadwell and Suzanne Sorrells. *Ostomy Management*, May/June 1979:3–5.
"Potassium Imbalance," *NCP Guide* #2:48, 2nd Ed., Nurseco, 1980.
"Promoting a Positive Sexual Adjustment Following Ostomy Surgery," by Karla Rose-Williamson. *Ostomy Management*, May/June 1979:11–16.
"Responses to Loss: the Grief and Mourning Process," *NCP Guide* #1:31, 2nd Ed., Nurseco, 1980.
Sex, Pregnancy and the Female Ostomate, Sex and the Male Ostomate, Ileostomy—A Guidebook, and other literature. United Ostomy Assn., Inc., 2001 Beverly Blvd., Los Angeles, CA 90057.
"Teaching Patients: General Suggestions," *NCP Guide* #1:49, 2nd Ed., Nurseco, 1980.
"Teaching Patients: Specific Plan for Skills and Procedures," *NCP Guide* #1:50, 2nd Ed., Nurseco, 1980.
"The Patient Experiencing a Body Image Disturbance," *NCP Guide* #2:29, 2nd Ed., Nurseco, 1980.

The Patient with a Mastectomy

Definition: Excision of a breast: simple (breast only) or radical (breast with extensive lymph node dissection in surrounding tissues).

LONG TERM GOAL: The patient will return to her optimum level of health and resume usual roles in home, family, community following a safe, successful breast removal and a suitable convalescence aimed at accepting her altered body image and loss; the patient will express optimism, self-confidence and a desire to live life fully and wholly again.

General Considerations:

— **Incidence:** One in thirteen American women will develop breast cancer at some time in their life; over 100,000 new cases yearly, over 35,000 deaths yearly from breast cancer. More than 80% of lumps are first found by women themselves; most (over 80%) of these lumps are benign; high risk factors include previous cancer of breast and/or breast cancer in a close relative.

— **Cancer detection:** Nurses can assume an important role in early cancer detection by serving as specialized volunteers to teach breast self-examination in public health education programs. Training materials, films, and guidelines are readily available at the local ACS chapters. Nurses should remember and teach signs of possible breast cancer.

      B-breast mass, fixed, rigid, irregular;

      R-retraction, inverted nipple, "orange peel" skin signs;

      E-edema, swelling, change in size;

      A-axillary involvement of glands and nodes;

      S-sanguinous nipple discharge;

      T-tenderness.

— **Treatment:** Patients with breast disease are usually admitted for an excisional biopsy with frozen section and possible mastectomy. A simple lumpectomy may be indicated; a radical mastectomy may be needed, followed by (for metastases) radiation therapy, chemotherapy and/or hormonal therapy, oophorectomy, adrenalectomy, or hypophysectomy.

— **Preoperative nursing responsibilities** include:

    (1) Routine preop nursing care; refer to NCPG #2:44, "General Preoperative Nursing Care";

    (2) Specific teaching re: Hemovac, positioning, coughing and deep breathing exercises, dressing, pain relief & arm exercises;

    (3) Psychological and emotional care and counseling re: the information and reassurances that the patient needs and wants (hospitalization, the impending operation and probability of mastectomy, the postoperative course anticipated). Find out what the patient has been told and what is planned. Attempt to identify and resolve any distortions or misconceptions the patient may have. Do not force more information than the patient can tolerate or accept. Encourage patient to express her feelings and fears freely, even to cry. Normal and common fears include those of dying, of cancer, of disfigurement, of loss of sexuality, and of pain.

(4) Preparation of the family (or significant other), i.e. providing information, encouraging them to express their concerns and questions, helping them to understand the patient's feelings.

— **Postoperative nursing responsibilities** include:

(1) Routine postop nursing care; refer to NCPGs #2:41, 42, 43, "General Postoperative Nursing Care, Part A, Part B, Part C";

(2) Care of incision and arm: positioning, drainage, dressings; see below and refer to your hospital and surgeon's protocol;

(3) Psychological and emotional care to accept body image change and loss of breast as well as diagnosis of cancer with its implications; refer to NCPG #1:31, "Responses to Loss; the Grief and Mourning Process," and NCPG #2:29, "Body Image Disturbance."

(4) Teaching re: arm exercises, breast self-examination, prostheses and clothing selection; see below and refer to your own hospital's patient education program for mastectomy or develop one yourself in collaboration with American Cancer Society representative. Some of the information about prostheses and clothing will need to be provided by out-patient clinic or office nurse, by public health or visiting nurse, and/or by ACS volunteers in the weeks and months following the patient's discharge. The hospital staff nurse should be armed with referral names and numbers, with the addresses of local department stores or mastectomy boutiques that are prepared to help patient, and with literature on prostheses to use if requested.

— **Reach to Recovery Volunteers** are 3 years postop mastectomy patients verified by two doctors as being physically healed and psychologically adjusted. With the patient's physician request, the volunteer will visit in hospital or at home, bringing a kit of supplies, useful information, friendship, and strict confidentiality, free of charge.

— **The YWCA ENCORE National Program**, est. 1975, entails free, weekly group meetings of mastectomy patients for 30 min. "land exercises" and 30 min. "water therapy exercises" (shallow end of pool). A written consent form from the doctor is necessary.

Specific Considerations, Potential Patient Outcomes, and Nursing Actions:

1) General Surgery Postop Measures

The patient will resume normal cardio/pulmonary/renal functions; fluid and electrolyte balance will be maintained and elimination patterns restored; the patient will be free of preventable complications:
— refer to NCPGs #2:41, 42, & 43;
— administer antibiotics, vitamin/mineral supplements, sedatives, etc. as ordered, observing & reporting untoward reactions;
— give fluids & food as tolerated when peristalsis returns;
— watch for bladder distention & constipation; take corrective measures needed.

2) Rest and Comfort

The patient will experience reduced discomfort and pain, less tension on the suture line; will be free of preventable immobility; the patient will maintain adequate ventilation, have clear lungs and will cough up bronchial secretions:
— position on back or unaffected side in semi-Fowler's position; use pillows & towels as cushions to keep elbow higher than shoulder, hand higher than elbow, joints flexed in functional position;
— turn, cough & deep breathe pt. Q2H, using gentle, firm support when moving affected arm; support chest during coughing;
— offer pain medication Q3-4H PRN; know that incisional pain lasts one to two weeks, but some pts. have intermittent pain or paresthesia at site for several weeks;

— give passive & active leg exercises Q4H until ambulatory; have pt. sit on side of bed, dangling legs with affected arm supported adequately for comfort; get pt. up to bathroom and begin progressive ambulation when surgeon permits.

3) Dressings & Drainage

The patient's incision will heal without infection or excessive bleeding; the patient will gradually assist with dressing changes until, by discharge, she can care for own wound site:

— observe & record amt. & kind of drainage: handle Hemovac (or Vacu-Drain) & tubes carefully with aseptic technique; reinforce dressings as needed;

— report immediately excessive bleeding; check pulse & BP for significant change;

— encourage pt.'s acceptance & viewing of incisional site; gradually have pt. assist with dressing changes; teach pt. signs of infection to note & report to doctor, following discharge.

4) Arm Exercises

The patient's arm will be restored to full motion and usefulness; contractures, loss of function and stiffness will be controlled and muscle tone will be preserved:

— make referral for physical rehabilitation, if formal program for mastectomy pts. is available in your hospital;

— have ACS Reach to Recovery Volunteer come in to teach exercises, if surgeon requests this in writing;

— refer to NCPG #1:45, "Arm Exercises for the Mastectomy Patient"; explain & demonstrate each exercise;

— stay with pt. while she does them for the first few days; use the opportunity to provide information, reassurance, encouragement & to assess any problems or answer any questions;

— involve a family member or friend to assist in encouragement of pt. & to help ensure faithfulness to exercise program in the weeks & mos. following discharge.

5) Psychosocial Adjustment

The patient will adapt effectively to the trauma of surgery, to her loss of breast and altered body image, to a cancer diagnosis and to the stress of an intensive rehabilitation regimen; the patient will express feelings openly and will gradually feel more confident and able to cope:

— provide time to talk, to ask questions, to express feelings; remain with pt. for periods of time, even when pt. does not wish to talk; refer to NCPG #1:31 ". . . The Grief and Mourning Process;"

— allow the pt. to cry, to express anger, etc. in order to move steadily through grieving process without delay; help pt. to understand that crying spells, frightening dreams, helplessness & depression are not unusual & will pass;

— discuss her adjustment with family & friends; encourage them to support her attractiveness & self-worth; have them reassure the pt. that her femininity, sexuality & lovability are not affected by her appearance; help them to accept, to understand, & help pt.;

— consult surgeon re: information to be given pt. by whom; try to get a written request for a R-T-R Volunteer;

— teach pt. proper techniques of Breast Self-Examination; provide ACS pamphlet on topic (see references); help pt. accept fact that mastectomy pts. are higher risks & early detection of lump in other breast is her responsibility;

— accentuate the positive aspects of the pt.'s strengths, resources & value (to herself as well as others); identify & support the pt.'s desire to live fully again for as long as possible;

— evaluate emotional rehabilitation by time of discharge & make appropriate referrals for follow-up mental health care PRN; observe & assess pt. for signs of withdrawal, insomnia, depression, severe anxiety, helplessness & hopelessness.

Discharge Planning and Teaching Objectives/Outcomes

1) (Patient/Family/Significant Other) Has been given a booklet or list of arm exercises and can demonstrate them accurately. Knows she should continue them for four to six months.

2) Has been given a pamphlet on Breast Self-Examination and can correctly demonstrate technique. Knows she must do this once monthly between periods, or at regular intervals.

3) Knows how to care for incisional area, dressings, etc. Knows what signs of infection (redness, swelling, increased drainage, odor, fever) to note and report promptly to doctor. Knows that complete healing should occur before fitting for a permanent prosthesis.

4) Knows that physical and mental exhaustion, probably related to stress reaction, will linger for several weeks; nevertheless, social visits and resumption of activities of daily living should be gradually undertaken.

5) States she knows how to prevent lymphedema (or swollen arm): sleeping or sitting with affected arm elevated; keeping skin clean, healthy, free of injuries and minor infections; using talcum powder instead of anti-perspirants which clog pores; exercising arm faithfully; refraining from using tight bracelets or carrying heavy handbags or packages; wearing gloves for house and yard work; and avoiding extremes of heat or cold.

Recommended References

"Arm Exercises for the Mastectomy Patient," *NCP Guide* #1:45, 2nd. Ed., Nurseco, 1980.

"Breast Cancer: Confronting One's Changed Image," a series of articles by various authors. *American Journal of Nursing*, September 1977:1430–1436.

"Breast Cancer—Helping the Mastectomy Patient Live Life Fully," by Joanne Tully and Beatrice Wagner. *Nursing 78*, January 1978:18–25.

"Breast Examination Practices," by Ellie Turnbull. *American Journal of Nursing*, September 1977:1450, 1451.

"Breast Self-Examination," by Doris Burger. *American Journal of Nursing*, June 1979:1088, 1089.

Breast Self-Examination, Reach To Recovery (pamphlets for patients). American Cancer Society, Inc., 521 W. 57th St., New York, NY 10019.

"General Postoperative Nursing Care, Part A, B, & C," *NCP Guides* #2:41, 42, 43, 2nd. Ed., Nurseco, 1980.

"General Preoperative Nursing Care," *NCP Guide* #2:44, 2nd. Ed., Nurseco, 1980.

"Responses to Loss: the Grief and Mourning Process," *NCP Guide* #1:31, 2nd. Ed., Nurseco, 1980.

"The Patient Experiencing a Body Image Disturbance," *NCP Guide* #2:29, 2nd. Ed., Nurseco, 1980.

The Patient with a Peptic Ulcer
(Medical Management)

Definition: A "peptic" ulcer is an erosion of the digestive lining by pepsin and hydrochloric acid. Included in this classification are gastric and duodenal ulcers, plus the relatively rare esophageal and jejunal ulcers.

LONG TERM GOAL: The patient will achieve an optimum level of functioning within a modified lifestyle and a therapeutic regimen needed to get ulcer healed and to prevent recurrences.

General Considerations:

— **Signs and Symptoms:** Gnawing, burning, mid-epigastric pain occurring 2-4 hrs. after eating & relieved by food or antacids. Nausea, bloating, heartburn, belching, changes in bowel habits or weight are common complaints. Hematemesis and/or tarry stools may be present.

— Duodenal ulcers are associated with excessive secretions of HCl acid while gastric ulcers are commonly caused by injury associated with various drugs, chemicals or bile reflux. Most (about 80%) ulcers are located in the duodenum and, of these, nearly all are benign. Malignancy is more often seen in patients with gastric ulcers but still the percentage is small. Diagnostic tests to rule out cancer are nearly always done. Gastric analysis, upper GI x-rays, fiberoptic panendoscopy supplement the usual lab work.

— Surgery is usually not required for most ulcer patients. See NCPG #1:16, "The Patient with a Peptic Ulcer (Surgical Management)."

— **Medical treatment** consists of rest, diet, and medications designed to obtain the following expected outcomes:
(1) Healing of ulcer within two to six weeks;
(2) Relief of pain and epigastric discomfort promptly;
(3) Prevention of complications requiring surgical intervention;
(4) Reduction of motor and secretory activity of the stomach and duodenum;
(5) Correction of any systemic imbalances to improve the general health status;
(6) Acceptance of ulcer diagnosis and willingness to follow treatment plan in order to prevent recurrences.

— **Nursing responsibilities** include (1) assessment, care, and evaluation activities to promote effective healing of the patient's ulcer; and (2) counseling and teaching activities to enable the patient to understand and accept an appropriate therapeutic regimen and modified lifestyle to prevent recurrence of ulcer.

Specific Considerations, Potential Patient Outcomes, and Nursing Actions:

1) Rest and Comfort, Relaxation

The patient will experience physical and mental rest in a tension-reduced atmosphere; the patient's stress reduction will produce lessened gastric/duodenal spasm and secretion of acid:
— reduce light, noise, unwelcome visitors & unnecessary stimuli in surroundings;
— turn periodically & position for comfort, encouraging short napping sessions throughout the day;
— give back rubs & use muscle relaxation techniques to reduce tension; consider use of biofeedback, self-hypnosis, or transcendental meditation techniques to enable patient to induce his own state of relaxation;
— observe & record signs of anxiety, tension, restlessness or annoyance; attempt to eliminate or reduce stressors affecting pt.; use nursing care plan & conferences for a consistent nursing staff approach to pt. care;
— provide time to talk with & listen to the patient, demonstrating a warm, understanding interest & concern with his problems; help pt. to express feelings & to understand what & why certain situations & people irritate; explore the possible avenues of true relaxation relevant to pt., e.g. music, art, reading, hobbies, active exercise, sports, etc.; let pt. suggest changes that s/he wants to make to decrease stress;
— administer sedatives, tranquilizers & antispasmodics as frequently as ordered & on time; teach pt. purposes of each & ask him to help note effect, duration & untoward reactions; refer to NCPG #2:45, "Drugs: Hypnotics & Sedatives" & NCPG #2:47 "Drugs: Tranquilizers"; for anticholinergics note dry mouth, rapid pulse, increased blood pressure, difficulty swallowing, dry & flushed skin, blurred vision, constipation, urinary retention, or dizziness.

2) Diet/Antacid Therapy

The patient will experience pain relief; the gastric acidity will be reduced and neutralized; the stomach will be coated with non-absorbable buffering solution most of the time:
— give antacid medications as often as necessary & as ordered, usually every hour or two when awake & whenever pain arises;
— know & teach pt. that liquid antacids act faster than tablets, although tablets are more convenient to carry; use three tablets to equal 1 tablespoon of liquid antacid & remind pt. to chew tablets to hasten absorption; both are taken with a full glass of water;
— observe elimination to note antacid effects of constipation, diarrhea, renal dysfunction or electrolyte imbalance;
— warn pts. never to substitute one brand of antacid for another without doctor's permission; the differing health needs of pt. & the differing effects of various antacids make the specific selection a deliberate decision & responsibility of MD;
— give six, small, bland feedings of diet as ordered; usually it is low fiber (no raw fruits or vegetables), moderate protein & fat, & lacking in strong spices or foods that cause the particular pt. distress; coffee (reg. *or* decaf.), tea, cola & chocolate are to be avoided; milk substitutes, low sodium preparations, dietary preferences & other special needs should be considered & the pt. should be actively involved in the planning & selection of appropriate foods; include the family in dietary teaching.

3) Prevention of Complications
: Systemic imbalances caused by past or present health problems will be prevented and corrected; complications of intractibility, hemorrhage, obstruction and perforation will be prevented or promptly identified and controlled:
— observe & report signs of hematemesis, tarry stools, 20 mm. drop in BP, rapid pulse, pallor, diaphoresis, weakness, chills, restlessness, possible hyperventilation, or sudden & severe upper abdominal pain & rigidity; notify MD STAT and perform standard nursing orders for control of hypovolemic shock (IV,0_2, NG tube, lab work);
— know & teach pt. that smoking is discouraged because nicotine decreases the bicarbonate content of pancreatic juice which helps neutralize gastric acid & because smoking delays ulcer healing;
— encourage & support pt. in decisions to eliminate smoking, alcohol, aspirin & long working hours or other stress producing elements insofar as possible; reinforce healthy behaviors, but leave responsibility with the pt. & family; ;
— assess pt.'s needs & resources for utilizing community health personnel, e.g. school nurse, industrial nurse, mental health counselors & self-help growth groups; make referrals PRN.

Discharge Planning and Teaching Objectives/Outcomes

1) (Patient/Family/Significant Other) Can state basic facts re: ulcer, causes, treatment, signs and symptoms of complications; knows where own ulcer is and influencing factors.
2) Has general outline of doctor's recommendations regarding work and rest patterns, need to avoid smoking, alcohol, caffeine, aspirin and other stress-producing, acid-causing elements in own life. States s/he understands importance of continuing regimen throughout the healing period until MD tapers off the treatment.
3) Has received, read and knows written instructions re: antacids, tranquilizers, anti-spasmodics and other medications s/he is to take; can state dosage, frequency, desired effects and untoward symptoms to be reported to doctor.
4) Has received, read and can give dietary instructions; can plan a typical day's menu and tell what is permitted and disallowed on diet. Agrees to eat small, frequent feedings to avoid hungry state. States s/he knows that s/he should avoid both regular and decaffeinated coffee, cola drinks, tea, chocolate as well as highly seasoned foods, raw fruits and vegetables and specifically those foods that cause a problem for self.
5) Has identification card for wallet with name, address, diagnosis, drugs and dosage, blood type and doctor's name and phone number.

Recommended References
"Drugs: Hypnotics & Sedatives," *NCP Guide* #3:45. Nurseco, 1977.
"Drugs: Tranquilizers," *NCP Guide* #3:47, Nurseco, 1977.
"The Patient with a Peptic Ulcer (Surgical Management)," *NCP Guide* #1:16, 2nd Ed., Nurseco, 1980.
"What to Teach Your Patient About His Duodenal Ulcer," by Joan Kratzer and Dorothy Rauschenberger. *Nursing 78*, January 1978:54,55.

The Patient with a Peptic Ulcer
(Surgical Management)

Definitions: **Gastrectomy** is removal of the stomach; it may be total or subtotal (more common).
Vagotomy is cutting the vagal nerve to the stomach to diminish neural stimulation of gastric secretion; results also in diminished motility of stomach and intestine with a delayed stomach emptying time; may be **selective** to preserve hepatic and biliary branches or **superselective** to preserve innervation of pyloric sphincter while denervating only parietal cell mass.
Pyloroplasty is the procedure in which drainage is improved by slitting the pylorus longitudinally and sewing it to the bottom of the stomach for another exit.
Antrectomy is removal of the distal third of the stomach which secretes the hormone gastrin, a gastric secretion stimulant.
Gastroduodenostomy (Bilroth I) is an antrectomy with anastomosis of the remainder of the stomach to the duodenum.
Gastrojejunostomy (Bilroth II) is removal of most of the stomach and anastomosis of the stump to the jejunum.

LONG TERM GOAL: The patient will recover from a safe, successful gastric resection of his ulcer; the patient will return to usual roles in home, family, community after a normal, short convalescence.

General Considerations:
— **C-H-O-P:** Chronicity (intractibility), Hemorrhage, Obstruction, Perforation: these are the four indications for gastric resection of an ulcer. The type of operation depends on the site of the ulcer and the situation to be corrected. Often a combination of the above mentioned procedures is done.
— **Nursing responsibilities:** Preoperatively, the care is similar to those having general abdominal surgery. Refer to NCPG #2:44, "General Preoperative Care," for assessment of patient and suggestions for teaching. When surgery is elective and time allows, much important information may be transmitted. Even if patient status is deteriorating and surgery is imminent, provide some time to answer patient/family questions and assuage fears. A nasogastric tube is placed, a standard abdominal skin prep is completed, continuous intravenous fluids are given and a CVP Line is placed. Refer to NCPG #2:46, "Intravenous Therapy," and #2:40, "Central Venous Pressure Line."

Specific Considerations, Potential Patient Outcomes, and Nursing Actions:
1) CardiopulmonaryThe patient will maintain adequate ventilation; the patient coughs up bronchial secretions; the patient has clear lungs and is
   Function   free of atelectasis and pneumonia; the patient has efficient circulating blood volume and complications of hemorrhage and shock are prevented/controlled:
   — refer to NCPG #2:41, Part A: "Support of Pulmonary Functions," & NCPG #2:42, Part B: "Support of Cardiovascular/ Renal Functions";

— turn, cough & deep breathe pt. Q2H; IPPB treatments are given to stimulate deep breathing & mucus removal; give pain medication 30 min. before treatments; cover incision with pillow & hands to support incision before coughing; teach pt./ family importance of doing this; observe pt. closely after IPPB for change of status;
— check CVP & record hourly; monitor & record TPR & BP as ordered, noting quality & changes;
— check dressing for bleeding; reinforce as necessary; keep MD informed.

2) Fluid and Electrolytes

The patient maintains an optimum fluid and electrolyte balance; the patient has a satisfactory intake and output; the patient is free of preventable complications and imbalances:
— accurately monitor & record all fluid intake & output, carefully measuring solution used to irrigate NG tube; estimate diaphoresis & wound drainage; gastric suction & urine measurements should be exact;
— observe for fluid & electrolyte imbalance; refer to NCPGs #3:48 & 3:49, "Fluids & Electrolytes, Part A: Fluids, Part B: Electrolytes";
— keep nasogastric tube patent, functioning & securely connected to low, intermittent suction; don't try to push, pull or reposition tube to avoid injury to gastric suture line; irrigate tube with prescribed amt. of NS as often as ordered & needed, recording amt. used & returned on I & O record; note color & amt. of drainage (should be bright red turning to dark red after first 12-24 hrs. post-op); report excessive bleeding & vomiting immediately;
— lubricate nostrils & give oral hygiene Q3H; topical anesthetic sprays may provide temporary relief of sore throat;
— clamp NG tube when ordered; give prescribed amt. water every hour; discontinue & reconnect tube if pt. becomes distended, nauseated or vomits; if well tolerated, aspirate residual gastric contents in 4 hrs.; record amt. & notify MD; check for returning bowel sounds by auscultation of abdomen & by asking pt. if s/he has passed flatus;
— when NG tube removed, give clear to full liquid diet in small amts.; then advance to soft, bland diet in six small daily feedings;
— observe for signs of "dumping syndrome" (diaphoresis, abdominal cramping, weakness, flushing, increased pulse) & have pt. lie down for 30 min. after meals; explain phenomenon & teach pt. to take only a very small amt. fluids with meals & to avoid sweet, high CHO meals for six mos. or until new sized stomach can adapt;
— early post-op, foley catheter will be in place for accurate output measurement & prevention of complications; after removal, check voiding & urine specific gravity & appearance;
— administer parenteral fluids, observing administration site for redness, infiltration, leakage;
— check bowel elimination; report diarrhea or constipation; take corrective measures.

3) Control of Infection

The patient will be free of infections:
— note & report temperature elevations of two or more degrees 3rd PO Day;
— administer antibiotics ordered with appropriate methods for effectiveness, checking literature & pharmacist;
— use strict aseptic technique when handling dressings, drainage tubes & collection devices.

4) Comfort Measures & Psychosocial Adjustment	The patient will adapt effectively to trauma of surgery and the stress of hospitalization; the patient and family will experience relief of fears and pain and will express feelings of growing strength and independence:

— administer analgesics liberally first 48 hrs. postop & after that PRN, remembering individual needs & pain thresholds;

— change position regularly; perform passive and active range of motion exercises; see NCPG #1:47 "Range of Motion Exercises"; progress to increasing ambulation, checking pulse & BP before & after sitting or walking;

— refer to NCPG #2:43, "General Postop Care, Part C: Support of Auxiliary Functions";

— assess psychological status of pt. & refer to NCP Guides re: behaviors, #s1:20-33;

— as recovery progresses, explain to pt. & family what is happening, how pt. is progressing and what s/he needs & wants to know to prepare for discharge.

Discharge Planning and Teaching Objectives/Outcomes

1) (Patient/Family/Significant Other) Has written appointment date and time for follow-up visit with doctor; knows to seek medical attention for any signs of infection, unexplained persistent discomfort and nutritional difficulties (digestion disorder or weight loss) that may arise.

2) State s/he knows what to do about "dumping syndrome" (which *may* occur), i.e. avoid high carbohydrate meals, take fluids with meals, & remember to lie down after meals.

3) Knows what to expect re: convalescence: gradual, moderate exercise for six weeks; diet as tolerated but in small amounts several times daily; care of suture line (soap & water cleansing, dry, sterile dressing).

4) Has received, read and can give written instructions re: antacids, tranquilizers, vitamins and other medications (analgesics, hynotics) s/he is to take; can state dosage, frequency, desired effects and untoward symptoms to be reported to doctor.

Recommended References

"Central Venous Pressure Line," *NCP Guide* #2:40, 2nd Ed., Nurseco, 1980.

"Fluids & Electrolytes, Part A: Fluids, Part B: Electrolytes," *NCP Guides* #3:48, 49, Nurseco, 1977.

"General Preoperative Nursing Care," *NCP Guide* #2:44, 2nd Ed., Nurseco, 1980.

"General Postoperative Nursing Care, Part A: Support of Pulmonary Functions, Part B: Support of Cardiovascular/Renal Functions, & Part C: Support of Auxiliary Functions," *NCP Guides* #2:41, 42, 43, 2nd Ed., Nurseco, 1980.

"Intravenous Therapy: General Principles," *NCP Guide* #2:46, 2nd Ed., Nurseco, 1980.

The Patient with Pneumonia

Definition: Inflammation of the pulmonary air sacs with resultant filling of the alveoli with an exudate.

LONG TERM GOAL: The patient will recover from pneumonia without complications, able to resume usual life roles (define the usual roles).

General Considerations:
— Pneumonia is the **fifth leading cause of death**, especially in the very young and elderly. It is often seen co-existing with another disease, commonly alcoholism or influenza. When combined with the latter, it is the leading cause of death in infectious diseases.
— **The causative organisms** are around us all the time and are carried by droplet infection or contact with infected persons/carriers. Pneumonia generally occurs when body resistance is lowered, when a person is exposed to a large concentration of organisms or to particularly virulent ones, or by any bronchial obstruction associated with mucus formation.
— Every patient on bed rest is a **potential candidate** for hypostatic pneumonia, thus frequent turnings are essential to prevent pooling of the secretions.
— **Nursing responsibilities** include assessing the patient's current health status, prescribing nursing interventions, providing drug therapy as ordered, and teaching the patient/family/significant other good general health maintenance and disease prevention.

Specific Considerations, Potential Patient Outcomes, and Nursing Actions:

1) Respiratory Function

The patient will maintain a patent airway; the patient will raise and expectorate pulmonary secretions; the patient will regain adequate pulmonary ventilation:
— keep head of bed elevated; place pt. on side with one pillow lengthwise to support entire back & help expand chest;
— turn Q1-2H; have pt. cough & try to raise mucus at least Q1H; splint painful part of pt.'s chest with your hands to minimize pain; mucus should be expectorated into tissues, not swallowed; if pt. unable to raise mucus on own, suction PRN; do cough routine ½ hour after giving pain medication;
— assist with IPPB & postural drainage PRN: prevent smoking in room, even if pt. not on O_2;
— explain cause of dyspnea to pt. and the expected outcome (that s/he should feel better in 24-72 hours).

2) Pain, Rest and Comfort

The patient will be free of severe pleuretic pain; the patient will experience only minimal anxiety associated with condition; the patient will maintain an adequate rest pattern:
— give analgesics & sedatives as ordered but observe for depressed respirations;
— provide fluids, turnings, coughings, back & mouth care, etc. all at same time so pt. can rest in-between;
— check linens for dampness (from perspirations) & change PRN; prevent pt. from chilling;

— assess anxieties & fear; normal ones are those of choking, dying; tell pt. you will be checking on him at least Q½H to observe his breathing;

— know that abd. & front shoulder pain often accompany early pneumonia; explain to pt. & reassure they will subside;

— know & explain to pt. that coughing up blood is common after the first few days of unproductive coughing & does not mean that s/he is worse.

3) Fever and Hydration

The patient will regain a normal body temperature; the patient will maintain a normal fluid balance:

— check vital signs at least Q4H & PRN; provide cooling measures (sponges, etc.) for temperature over 102;

— give antibiotics on time in order to maintain blood levels; watch for sensitivity;

— monitor skin, tongue, I&O for signs of dehydration; refer to NCPGs #3:48 & 49, "Fluids and Electrolytes, Parts A and B";

— record I&O; fluid loss will be high from fever, dehydration, dyspnea, & diaphoreses; ensure a high fluid intake within limits of pt.'s cardiac reserve.

4) Prevention of Complications

The patient will be free of preventable complications:

— know that two common complications are abdominal distention & paralytic ileus (watch for gaseous distention, tense abdomen, dull & diffuse pain, depressed peristalsis, infrequent bowel sounds, vomiting after meals); assess for adequate urinary output & daily BM; know that other complications are pleural effusion, lung abscess, sustained hypotension & shock, meningitis, congestive heart failure;

— restlessness may preclude delirium; withhold sedatives & check with Dr.; monitor carefully pts. with alcoholism or any chronic pulmonary problems; assess changes in mental status, behavior, or stupor; see NCPG #4:41, "Assessment of Mental Status."

Discharge Planning and Teaching Objectives/Outcomes

1) (Patient/Family/Significant Other) Can obtain assistance with meals, etc. PRN; knows to resume daily activities very gradually.

2) Understands the importance of avoiding overexertion, fatigue, chilling, exposure to crowds, air pollution, and persons with infections; knows that state of lowered resistance lasts for a considerable time. Promises to practice deep breathing exercises 3X daily, during convalescence.

3) Knows what medications to take and when, as well as why.

4) Realizes necessity of keeping follow-up Dr.'s appointment, even if feeling better.

Recommended References

"Assessment of Mental Status." *NCP Guide* #4:41, Nurseco, 1978.

"Fluids and Electrolytes, Part A: Fluids." *NCP Guide* #3:48, Nurseco, 1977.

"Fluids and Electrolytes, Part B: Electrolytes." *NCP Guide* #3:49, Nurseco, 1977.

"Your Patient's Second Threat?" by Carol M. Taylor, RN, MS. *Nursing '76*, March 1976:30–38.

The Patient with Rheumatoid Arthritis

Definition: RA is a chronic, systemic, inflammatory disease affecting the synovium, causing painful, unstable joints and serious, crippling deformities; each successive exacerbation causes more tissue damage; remissions can last months or years.

LONG TERM GOAL: The patient will reach the highest level of functioning within the chronic limitations of arthritis; the patient will perform activities of daily living with confidence, self-esteem and a measure of independence; the patient will accept and comply cooperatively with a comprehensive treatment and rehabilition program for as long as needed.

General Considerations:
— **Incidence:** Occurs in about 3% of the population, most commonly in the 40s; women affected three times more than men in age group of 25-45.
— **Signs and Symptoms:** Morning stiffness for ½ hr. to several hours, fatigue, weight loss, malaise & warm, tender, swollen joints, eventually becoming distorted and subluxated; mild anemia & elevated erythrocyte sedimentation rate.
— **Aims of treatment:**
  (1) control of pain and reduction of inflammation;
  (2) prevention and correction of joint damage and deformities;
  (3) attainment of best possible mobility and function;
  (4) self-sufficient performance of ADL; and
  (5) improvement in activity tolerance (more stamina).
— Most patients can be helped with treatment. About 10-15% of patients will need more radical treatment, including surgery, and newer investigational drugs or gold therapy (chrysotherapy).
— **Full treatment** includes: local and systemic rest balanced with exercise and activity; drug therapy; physical therapy (heat, massage, whirlpool, exercises); coordinated intensive rehabilitation (vocational, emotional, physical and social).
— **Nursing responsibility** rests primarily in patient/family education and counseling assistance of the patient through psychosocial adjustment and rehabilitation.

Specific Considerations, Potential Patient Outcomes, and Nursing Actions:
1) Rest and   The patient will maintain functional positions and optimum joint mobility, will have joint inflammation, muscle spasm, and pain
   Exercise   relieved, and will have further joint injury and deformity prevented:
                — during painful exacerbation phase, provide more rest with joints in functional alignment; when pain is controlled, provide necessary exercise & activity; a balance is important as too much rest causes stiffening, too much exercise causes

damage; frequent rest periods are needed to alleviate fatigue, but increased activity is needed to improve stamina; inactivity breeds discouragement, depression & further inactivity, then enormous efforts are required to restore acceptable activity levels;

— teach pt./family good body alignment & correct posture (sitting, standing & walking as well as light lifting); use foot boards, trochanter rolls, pillows & sandbags to maintain correct position;

— remember to pad & carefully apply aluminum or plastic splints, removable plaster casts & other supportive devices; keep underneath skin clean, dry, massaged & protected from pressure; observe periodically;

— apply soft, absorbent foot socks & gloves for warmth; consider elastic stockings PRN to support circulation;

— protect safety of pt. with trapeze, side rails, good wheelchairs, sturdy walkers, etc.; have pt. wear own shoes when walking, not soft-soled slippers; get adequate help when moving heavy or severely dependent pts.;

— consult with physical therapy for ways to reinforce & coordinate efforts: e.g. give analgesics before PT sessions, provide mental & emotional rest before & after therapy; assist with the assessment of functional abilities & physical activity tolerance levels; observe, when possible, exercise regimen & reinforce teaching; evaluate & help document increased strength & range of motion.

2) Drug Therapy   The patient will experience relief of pain as well as tissue and joint inflammation; the patient will verbalize awareness of medication effectiveness and untoward symptoms which need to be reported to physician:

— know that the usual dose of ASA is three 0.3 gm. tab. QID to achieve a salicylate blood level of 10-25 mg/100 ml., but then dosage is adjusted upward to control pt. symptoms of pain & swelling; observe & record reaction & tolerance; convince pt. to continue drug for its anti-inflammatory action, even if pain is lessened; teach pt. to take least expensive brand ASA available & to take it with meals, milk or antacids; ask pt. to report tarry stools, increasing stomach irritation, tinnitus (hearing loss of high pitched sounds);

— when giving NSAID (non steroid anti-inflammatory drugs eg. ibuprofen: Motrin, phenylbutazone: Butazolidin, indomethacin: Indocin, fenoprofen: Nalfon, oxyphenbutazone: Tandearil), give with meals, milk or antacid; monitor pt.'s weight, CBC; teach pt. to observe & report headaches, dizziness, visual disturbances, rash gastrointestinal distress & tarry stools; tarry stools;

— if giving corticosteroids, gold compounds or cytotoxic drugs, observe closely for serious toxic effects; review CBC & urinalysis reports for eosinophilia, hematuria, proteinuria & consult with Dr. regarding significant findings; record I & O, daily weight, vital signs; observe & report ulcerations of mouth & tongue or skin rashes & itching; use a flow sheet record form to make quick comparisons of significant data.

3) Psychosocial Adjustment & Rehabilitation	The patient will adjust adaptively to a serious, chronic disease which involves pain, limited capability, an uncertain future and some loss of independence; the patient will cooperatively participate in an intensive rehabilitation program:

— with pt./family/friends, discuss & clarify beliefs, attitudes & information about RA (i.e. danger of delaying treatment, misconceptions re: effectiveness of diet, climate, copper bracelets, "buckeye" or chestnut seed in pocket, etc.);

— explore common pt. fears of pain, crippling, loss of independence & frustration over other's lack of understanding & acceptance;

— share pt.'s experience of pain, listening for clues to alleviation; let pt. cooperatively plan own schedule, as far as possible, for medications, physical therapy, rest periods; refer to NCPG #1:30, "The Patient Experiencing Pain";

— know that emotional upsets & tension make condition worse; share this with pt. & together identify & attempt to alleviate causes of stress; discuss new & alternate methods of dealing with tension, e.g. swimming, use of a home jacuzzi, or hatha yoga classes can provide double benefits of therapeutic physical exercise along with emotional relaxation;

— assess what affect arthritis has on pt.'s self-concept; what activities does your pt. enjoy most, which are being hampered? how can they be modified so they may still be enjoyed? what are this pt.'s basic drives, needs, values? how much are interpersonal relationships disturbed? after discussing these topics with pt., seek to obtain the family & friend's understanding, acceptance & assistance of the pt.; refer to NCPG #2:29, "The Patient Experiencing a Body Image Disturbance";

— assist pt. to perform basic ADL, assessing need for assitive devices & helping pt. to obtain & use them correctly; see NCPG #1:49, "Teaching Patients: General Suggestions," and NCPG #1:50, "Teaching Patients: Specific Plan for Skills and Procedures";

— assess need for referrals to psychologist, mental health clinic, social services, community health nursing services, vocational rehabilitation; consult with physician & follow-through with paperwork;

— if surgery (joint fusion, artificial joints, bone resection) is needed, explore pt.'s feelings about proposed surgery, possible outcome, family & work arrangements, etc.; support realistic decisions;

— give pt. Arthritis Foundation pamphlets to take home & read; inform pt. of Foundation's services (loan closet of equipment).

Discharge Planning and Teaching Objectives/Outcomes

1) (Patient/Family/Significant Other) Can explain in own words basic facts about rheumatoid arthritis (e.g. nature of disease, symptoms, aggravating factors, treatment program to control pain and disability).

2) Has received, read and discussed at least one of The Arthritis Foundation's pamphlets supplied by medical personnel ("*Arthritis—The Basic Facts*," "*Rheumatoid Arthritis—A Handbook For Patients*").
3) Can state purpose, action, side effects to be reported, prescribed dosage and administration of all medications prescribed. Indicates willingness to continue medication even when symptoms are alleviated.
4) Can correctly demonstrate range of motion and other prescribed exercises for home usage; demonstrates correct posture and body mechanics; verbalizes acceptance of physical limitations and a willingness to plan activities accordingly, minimizing fatigue, strain and pain while maximizing effectiveness of therapeutic regimen.
5) Has been provided with a written set of instructions re: diet, exercises, medications, use of self-help devices and has appointment for medical follow-up; has verbally expressed confidence and willingness to carry out recommendations.
6) Has been evaluated for assistance (financial, vocational, convalescent hospital or home health care) and appropriate referrals have been made to state and local agencies.
7) Has received information re: additional community resources and services; has at least one community health resource person's name and number (besides doctor) in order to get additional help and information.

Recommended References

"Advice to Arthritics: Keep Moving," by Madeline C. Schwaid. *American Journal of Nursing*, October 1978:1708–1709.

Arthritis—The Basic Facts, The Truth About Aspirin for Arthritis, and *Rheumatoid Arthritis—A Handbook for Patients*. The Arthritis Foundation, 1212 Avenue of the Americas, New York, NY 10036.

Arthrtis Manual for Allied Health Professionals, The Arthritis Foundation (address above).

Fashions for the People Who Need Specially Designed Clothes. Vocational Guidance and Rehabilitation Services, 2239 E. 55th St., Cleveland, OH 44103.

"Gold Therapy for Rheumatoid Arthritis," by Marie Spruck. *American Journal of Nursing*, July 1979:1246–1248.

"How the Nurse Practitioner Manages the Rheumatoid Arthritis Patient," by Vicki Brown-Skeers. *Nursing 79*, June 1979:26–35.

"Rheumatoid Arthritis—Picking the Right Nonsteroid Drug," by Joseph DiPalma. *RN*, December 1977:63–72.

"Teaching Patients: General Suggestions." *NCP Guide #1:49*, 2nd Ed., Nurseco, 1980.

"Teaching Patients: Specific Plan for Skills and Procedures." *NCP Guide #1:50*, 2nd Ed., Nurseco, 1980.

"The Patient Experiencing A Body Image Disorder," *NCP Guide #2:29*, 2nd Ed., Nurseco, 1980.

"The Patient Experiencing Pain," *NCP Guide #1:30*, 2nd Ed., Nurseco, 1980.

The Patient with a Thoracotomy

Definitions: Thoracotomy: An opening into the thorax or pleural cavity.
Pneumonectomy: Removal of an entire lung.
Lobectomy: Removal of a lobe of a lung.
Segmental
Resection: Removal of one or more segments of a lobe.

LONG TERM GOAL: The patient will recover from the surgery free of preventable complications.

General Considerations:
— Read NCPG #2:44, "General Pre-Op Care," and NCPGs #s 2:41, 42, 43, "General Post-Op Care."
— Most thoracotomies are done for lung cancer, traditionally more common in men with a long history of smoking. The incidence of lung cancer in women is catching up with that of men due to the increase in smoking among women, and threatens to replace cancer of the breast in frequency.
— Thoracotomies are also done on patients with non-malignant pulmonary disease, e.g., bronchiectasis, coccidioidomycosis, benign tumors. Patients with decreased pulmonary function are at greater post-op risk than those with adequate pulmonary function.
— **Nursing responsibilities** include pre-op teaching that is specific to the thoracotomy; post-operatively, they are maintenance of vital functions, monitoring patient for early signs of potential complications, and health teaching of patient and family.

Specific Considerations, Potential Patient Outcomes, and Nursing Actions:
1) Pre-Op Patient   The patient will practice coughing, deep breathing, and arm exercise routine that will be done post-operatively:
   Training
— ask pt. if s/he has any questions & provide answers; if you don't have the information s/he seeks, try to get it;
— explain rationale to pt. for the Q2H turnings, coughing & deep breathing routine; tell pt. that you will provide pain med. before these routines to minimize discomfort; show pt. how you will splint chest during coughing for first few PO days, then teach pt. to splint own chest with a pillow; explain & have pt. use blow bottles;
— explain to pt. what s/he can expect re: chest tubes, IPPB, portable chest x-rays, ambulation, pain & discomfort;
— demonstrate, & have pt. practice, arm exercises; explain rationale for doing them (to regain normal arm & shoulder movements); check with surgeon to use this routine (exercise arm on operative side):
   a) start with arm at side, raise it straight up & try to touch head of bed;
   b) with arm at side, bend elbow, raise arm up to head & try to touch ear on opposite side of head;
   c) with elbow bent, raise arm up & out to shoulder level; try to bend hand back to touch pillow, forward to touch bed.

2) Respiratory Function The patient will maintain a patent airway and expand lung(s) adequately:
— elevate head of bed 30°-45° when BP is stabilized;
— turn pt. at least Q2H to back & *operative* side only (to ensure proper expansion of non-operative lung);
— if chest tube is in place, & when positioning pt. on side, place a towel on either side of tube, between pt. & bed (to keep tube from kinking & to minimize pt. discomfort);
— at each turning (Q2H), have pt. cough, use blow bottles, take deep breaths & try to raise sputum; to assist pt. with this, splint pt.'s chest on operative side with your hands or have patient splint with small pillow; use cupping & vibration techniques; give pain med. 20-30″ before coughing, turning, etc.
— suction sputum PRN until pt. has enough strength to expectorate it; know that one effect of surgery is to increase sputum production, & that it must be raised in order to avoid atelectasis;
— observe for signs of an ineffective cough & impending atelectasis (increased pulse, skin pallor);
— assess rate & quality of respirations; listen for lung sounds & report diminished breath sounds, rales & ronchi;
— be alert to signs of respiratory distress (increased dyspnea, cyanosis, sudden chest pain, lg. amt. of bleeding (more than 100cc's/H) into chest bottles); notify Dr. at once;
— watch for signs of abdominal distention which may push up the diaphragm & interfere with breathing;
— read NCPG #1:34 on care & maintenance of chest tubes;
— when pt. permitted to take fluids, know that warm ones will aid expectoration of mucus;
— know that excessive medication can depress respirations; medicate wisely so that respirations are not adversely affected but pt. is not in acute pain or discomfort.

3) Rest, Exercise, and Comfort The patient will rest and sleep between Q2H routine; will regain usual range of motion & function of arm, shoulder and trunk on operative side:
— do Q2H turning, coughing, etc. routine all at once so pt. may rest in-between;
— observe pt. for non-verbal signs of pain (anxiety, impaired sleep, restlessness, facial expressions, body position in bed); medicate PRN; give med. judiciously: enough to eliminate the acute pain but not depress respirations;
— keep head of bed elevated; place pillow at pt.'s back when positioned on side, plus one between legs;
— as soon as pt. is able, dangle on bed (at same time as turnings, etc.);
— start arm exercises 1st P.O. day, if OK with surgeon; pt. may need some assistance the first few times until his strength returns, or may use unaffected arm to lift other one during exercises; exercises should be DC'ed if pain & fatigue occur;
— when able to ambulate to bathroom and/or sit in chair, ensure safety & maintenance of chest tube & drainage bottle; *never* allow drainage bottle to go above level of pt.'s chest (or contents will run into pt.'s chest);
— share with pt./family, any signs of progress; explain role of equipment to family PRN.

Discharge Planning and Teaching Objectives/Outcomes

1) (Patient/Family/Significant Other) Knows what to expect in terms of fatigue, return of usual strength (fatigue & weakness for first 3 weeks is usual), and importance of rest and exercise in daily routine.
2) Knows the importance of continuing arm and shoulder exercises in order to maintain good functioning of arm and shoulder on operated side.
3) Knows what to expect in terms of change in pulmonary function, respiratory capacity and has a plan to adjust life style accordingly.
4) Has a supply of pain medication and knows how to obtain refills. Has a follow-up appointment with Dr./clinic.

Recommended References

"Bronchogenic Carcinoma: Pre-op and Post-op Care," by Sarah Cook, RN, MA. *RN*, September 1978:83–88, 90, 92, 94, 96.

"Chest Tubes and Bottles: Waterseal Drainage." *NCP Guide* #1:34, 2nd Ed., Nurseco, 1980.

"General Post-Op Care—Parts A, B, C." *NCP Guides* #s 2:41, 42, 43, 2nd Ed., Nurseco, 1980.

"General Pre-Op Care." *NCP Guide* #2:44, 2nd Ed., Nurseco, 1980.

"Treating Invasive Lung Cancer," by Marjorie W. Boyer. *American Journal of Nursing*, December 1977:1916–1923.

The Patient Manifesting Aggression

Definition: A forceful, attacking action, which may be physical, verbal or symbolic. It is unrealistic and directed toward the environment or inwardly toward the self.

LONG TERM GOAL: The patient will use realistic and self-protective (assertive) behavior to make known his needs and desires.

General Considerations:
— **Each aggressive incident should be reviewed** with a goal of improving patient care by identifying situations which contribute to aggression and by evaluating and revising interventions.
— **Nursing assessment** includes awareness of the behavioral manifestations of aggression which include:
  — overt, constant demands;
  — constant self-directed anger;
  — refusal to listen to staff;
  — constant or intermittent attempts at changing the plan of care;
  — abusive verbal language;
  — constant or intermittent non-adherence to Dr.'s orders.
— **Nursing responsibilities** include assessment of the patient's usual coping behaviors in order to recognize and support behaviors that are adaptive and positive.

Specific Considerations, Potential Patient Outcomes, and Nursing Actions:

1) Immediate Response to Recognition of Aggressive Behavior

The patient will limit or stop aggressive behavior:
— set limits on physically harmful behavior and explain to the pt. why you are doing so;
— contrast to the pt. his physical & emotional functioning that is realistic (assertive) versus that which is unrealistic and forceful (aggressive);
— always prepare the pt. (physically & verbally) for what you are going to do even if you consider it a daily and/or usual activity;
— encourage the pt. to express his feelings regarding the deprivation caused by the hospitalization & illness; sit down & listen; use open-ended questions;
— recognize that the pt.'s aggression may be in response to fear, increased dependency, &/or anxiety; therefore, do not attempt to defend yourself, the staff or the agency; listen to what the pt. is saying & assist him to understand his own method of coping.

| 2) Restoration to Adaptive Coping | The patient will utilize assertive behaviors as a means of expressing independence and control; will recognize and utilize outside sources of comfort and support: |

— know the difference between assertive (asking for what one wants; standing up for rights) and aggressive behavior (getting what one wants *at the expense of others*);

— plan the nursing care & daily routine with the pt., giving him as much flexibility in decision-making as possible; evaluate the care with him;

— reinforce positive (assertive) approaches utilized by the pt. ("I would like . . ." versus "Do this . . .");

— give the pt. the opportunity to plan & do things s/he likes to do, i.e. sleeping late, knitting, reading;

— praise the pt.'s efforts to maintain independence & be assertive;

— explain the reason for the pt.'s behavior to his significant others (SO), i.e., it is his way of coping;

— praise the efforts of the SOs in their attempts to assist the pt. in coping;

— stress to staff the importance of not chastising or rejecting the pt. for his efforts to cope by using aggressive behavior; rather, set limits on behavior that is physically destructive & teach the patient to be assertive instead of aggressive.

Discharge Planning and Teaching Objectives/Outcomes

1) (Patient/Family/Significant Other) Can verbalize behavior or demands that trigger the protective response of aggression.

2) Can describe the difference between assertiveness and aggression.

3) Can demonstrate at least one assertive behavior.

Recommended References

"Aggression as a Response," by Vallory G. Lathrop. *Perspectives in Psychiatric Care*, Sept.-Dec. 1978:202–205.

"Changing Behaviors: A Fun Approach that Works," by Kay M. Duffy. *RN*, December 1978:103–104.

"Mrs. Dowager: A Determinedly Disruptive Patient," by Mary T. Marks. *Nursing 73*, December 1973:17–19.

"The Violent Patient." *NCP Guide* #4:40, Nurseco, 1978.

"To Punish Herself, Laura Mutilated Her Body," by Karen R. Palermo. *Nursing 79*, June 1979:44–48.

"We Were No Match for 'Zorba the Greek'," by Darlene Rzepka. *Nursing 75*, September 1975:26–29.

The Patient Manifesting Anger

Definition: A strong feeling of displeasure, usually of antagonism.

LONG TERM GOAL: The patient will use realistic and self-protective (assertive) behavior to express his displeasure.

General Considerations:
— **Each angry outburst should be reviewed** with a goal of improving patient care by identifying situations which contributed to the outburst and by evaluating and revising interventions.
— **Nursing assessment** includes awareness of the behavioral manifestations of anger which include:
  — abusive verbal language;
  — constant negative verbalizations regarding hospital and staff;
  — refusal to participate in care;
  — refusal to eat or drink;
  — refusal to be dependent on staff;
  — throwing food or objects;
  — removal of treatment equipment from self (e.g. pulling out IV);
  — silence.
— **Nursing responsibilities** include assessment of the anger-provoking situation for cause and effect as well as assessment of the patient's usual coping behaviors in order to recognize and support those that are adaptive and positive.

Specific Considerations, Potential Patient Outcomes, and Nursing Actions:

1) Immediate Response to Recognition of Expressed Anger

The patient will eliminate the physically harmful and attacking expressions of anger; will express anger assertively rather than aggressively:
— tell the pt. you will prevent any further expression of anger that is physically harmful in nature;
— spend time with the pt.; ask him what the anger is about; if s/he refuses to answer, just sit with him while he is silent;
— praise any pt. efforts to put the anger into words & share the causes with you;
— be aware that a pt.'s anger is usually not meant for you personally, so do not respond defensively.

2) Restoration to Adaptive Coping

The patient will be able to discuss situations that provoke angry feelings; will be able to verbalize both positive and negative feelings related to angry outbursts:

— invite the pt. to participate in own care & to discuss feelings about the hospitalization;

— involve the pt. in own care on a continuing basis; ask him to do specific parts while you do others; discuss the results of this shared responsibility with him;

— continue to spend time daily conversing with the pt.; direct the conversation towards those aspects of the illness for which s/he has the most negative feelings; use open-ended questions;

— spend time with pt.'s significant others explaining pt.'s need to have the opportunity to express both positive & negative feeling about what is happening to him;

— praise the efforts of others to accept the conversational expressions by the pt. of his negative feelings;

— praise staff & family efforts to support the pt. & to understand the pt.'s behavior without personalizing it.

Discharge Planning and Teaching Objectives/Outcomes

1) (Patient/Family/Significant Other) Can verbalize behavior or demands that trigger the physically harmful aspects of patient's anger.

2) Can describe the difference between the conversational expression of anger and physically harmful/forceful behavior.

3) Can share both positive and negative feelings about an individual experience.

Recommended References

"Dealing with Rage." Nursing Grand Rounds. *Nursing 75*, October, 1975:24–29.

"Hostility," by Sister M. Martha Kiening in Carlson, Carolyn and Blackwell, Betty *Behavioral Concepts and Nursing Intervention*, 2nd ed., Philadelphia: J.B. Lippincott Co., 1978:128–140.

"Mr. O'Brien's Beard," by Rosemaire Hogan. *American Journal of Nursing*, January 1977:61.

"Privacy," by Dorothy W. Bloch in Carlson and Blackwell, *Behavioral Concepts and Nursing Interventions*, 2nd ed., Philadelphia: J.B. Lippincott, Co., 1978:226–239.

"The Staff Called Mrs. Jepson's Care Plan 'Resocialization.' I Called It a Repressive Regimen," by Joan Schuettler. *Nursing 74*, August 1974:10–12.

"The Violent Patient." *NCP Guide #4:40*, Nurseco, 1979.

"Understanding Anger," by Derry Ann Moritz. *American Journal of Nursing*, January 1978:81–83.

"We Should Have Been Tougher with Emma . . . and Ourselves," by Deborah Roediger. *Nursing 77*, May 1977:48–49.

The Patient Experiencing Anxiety

Definition: An uncomfortable feeling or tension which can be vague and/or intense. It occurs as a reaction to some unconscious threat that the person is experiencing.

LONG TERM GOAL: The patient will be able to use anxiety as a motivation for change and not be immobilized by it.

General Considerations:
— **Anxiety serves as a force** that warns the individual about threatening situations.
— **Nursing assessment** includes knowledge of the behavioral and physiological manifestations of anxiety which include:

Behavioral Manifestations		**Physiological Manifestations**	
— restlessness	— inability to retain information	— increased blood pressure	— dry mouth
— irritability	given	— rapid breath and pulse	— headaches
— rapid speech	— somatic complaints	— muscular tension	— nausea
— wringing of hands	— inability to communicate	— pounding heart	— dizziness
— repetitious questioning	— putting call light on frequently	— dilated pupils	— trembling
— inability to concentrate &/or	— disbelief of answers given	— perspiration	— cold, clammy hands
understand explanations		— gastric discomfort	

— **Nursing responsibilities** include assessment of the level of anxiety:
 (1) **mild anxiety:** alertness; an ability to recognize anxiety as a warning signal; learning can occur at this level;
 (2) **moderate anxiety:** selective inattention; a decreased ability to communicate or perceive the environment unless it is pointed out; learning can still occur at this level but it must be directed;
 (3) **severe anxiety:** a drastically reduced ability to perceive and communicate details; the whole is perceived but the connection between details cannot be made; learning cannot occur at this level;
 (4) **panic:** any detail which is perceived is elaborated and distorted; the person is unable to communicate or function; learning cannot take place.
— **Nursing interventions** should be directed toward the support and enhancement of those behaviors that are adaptive, positive and have assisted in resolving anxiety in past situations. In the panic level, the only successful interventions are those designed to make the person comfortable and reassured.

Specific Considerations, Potential Patient Outcomes, and Nursing Actions:

1) Immediate Response to Recognition of Anxious Behavior

The patient will be able to cope with the anxiety and reduce it at least one level:
— spend at least five minutes with the pt. TID & try to convey a willingness to listen & be supportive;
— encourage such coping mechanisms as talking, walking or crying;
— give the pt. clear, concise explanations of what is going to occur; repeat as often as necessary;
— do not overload the pt. with information; the pt. experiencing moderate to severe anxiety cannot retain or incorporate a great deal of data;
— do not make demands of the pt.;
— ask the pt. what you could do to make him feel more comfortable;
— if pt. hyperventilating, have pt. take slow, deep breaths; ask him to focus on how his body feels on expiration; breathe with pt. to give support;
— if pt. is in panic, stay with him, using physical touch PRN.

2) Restoration to Adaptive Coping

The patient will be able to identify sources of his anxiety:
— continue holding conversations with the pt.; increase the duration of each conversation but decrease the number of conversations per day;
— help pt. identify those tensions & environmental factors that create a feeling of anxiety;
— include the pt. in decisions about his care in order to create patient responsibility;
— give careful explanations of what will occur; ask the pt. for questions or concerns s/he may have about these events;
— encourage supportive family members to be patient since the pt. may not respond to them as before;
— praise staff & family members who are able to maintain an environment for the pt. that allows him to gain an understanding of & control over the anxiety.

Discharge Planning and Teaching Objectives/Outcomes
1) (Patient/Family/Significant Other) Can verbalize the way in which s/he copes with severe anxiety.
2) Can list environmental factors that elicit anxiety.
3) Can discuss ways of keeping patient responses to anxiety at a mild or moderate level and successfully cope with it.

Recommended References
"Drugs: Tranquilizers." *NCP Guide* #3:47, Nurseco, 1977.
"Effects of Hospitalization: Part A Tension Producing Causes." *NCP Guide* #1:40, 2nd Ed., Nurseco, 1980.
"Mrs. Kluska Wasn't Difficult . . . She Was Impossible," by Eileen Jahubek. *Nursing 77*, July 1977:36-37.
"Panic: Three Easy Steps to Restoring Control," by Sally Langendoen. *RN*, December 1978:44-47.
"The Patient Needing Crises Intervention." *NCP Guide* #2:31, 2nd Ed., Nurseco, 1980.
"Teaching a Concept of Anxiety to Patients," by Dorothea R. Hays. *Nursing Research*, Spring 1961:108-113.

The Patient Experiencing Confusion

Definition: A quality or state of being perplexed. It is the inability to comprehend and/or integrate words or events; may be of a temporary or permanent nature.

LONG TERM GOAL: The patient will be able to maintain touch with reality as much as possible.

General Considerations:
— **Confusion occurs** as a result of trauma, rapid change, infectious and metabolic disturbances, neurologic conditions, drug intoxication, cardiac and respiratory disturbances, and drug and alcohol withdrawal.
— **Nursing assessment** includes an awareness of the manifestations of confusion which include:
  — inability or vague identification of time, place, person;
  — appears drowsy most of the time;
  — decreased or no attention span;
  — recent memory is impaired;
  — inability to retain information given;
  — more confused at night than in daytime;
  — restless, aimless motions;
  — physical assault;
  — does not make eye contact for any period of time.
— **Nursing responsibilities** include assessment of the physiological state of functioning of the patient in order to differentiate between physiologically-induced confusion and psychologically and/or environmentally-induced confusion.
— **Nursing interventions** should reflect the causative factors. If the confusion is physiologically based, then nursing care must focus on the restoration of adaptive, physiological functioning; behavioral techniques can enhance the recovery but the basic physiological disturbance must be cleared up.

Specific Considerations, Potential Patient Outcomes, and Nursing Actions:

1) Immediate Response to Recognition of Confusion

The patient will recover from the physiologically or environmentally/psychologically-induced confusion and regain as much contact with reality as possible:
  — direct nursing care to the support of those physiological functions that are intact; give appropriate nursing care, & follow medical orders for treatment of the dysfunction;
  — always address the pt. by name & say who you are; the pt. may hear & understand you even if s/he does not acknowledge you;

— be consistent in informing the pt. what you are going to do; do not assume s/he is so confused that s/he will not understand;
— consistently involve the pt. in decision making & activity;
— reduce the amount of sensory overload/deprivation the pt. is experiencing: *for overload*: turn down lights or reduce noise of equipment; try to schedule nursing care activities so the pt. will have quiet times; *for deprivation*: have a staff member or another less confused pt. spend time with this pt., especially at mealtimes; seat the pt. with others or encourage familiar & positive visitors; whenever you are near the pt., touch him, say hello, bring pt. out of room into areas where s/he will have access to additional sensory stimuli;
— utilize appropriate safety measures to prevent injury to the pt. & others.

2) Restoration to Reality

The patient will maintain contact with reality as much as possible and will be aware of the need for assistance.
— praise the pt. for efforts at being with others & involved with the environment;
— be honest with the pt., don't just go along with his "reality," & don't encourage a denial of the confusion;
— avoid letting the pt. ramble, bring the conversation back to reality;
— use clear concise statements & questions; speak slowly & allow plenty of time for the pt. to answer; do not rush him;
— have pt. keep familiar objects with him, i.e., clock, own sleepwear, pictures of family, friends;
— have family members or friends share "old times" with the pt.;
— support & praise the pt.'s efforts to maintain conversation & reality-oriented behavior, encourage staff & the family to praise pt. for these efforts.

Discharge Planning and Teaching Objectives/Outcomes
1) (Patient/Family/Significant Other) Can identify time, place and person and is able to maintain a conversation that is indicative of being in touch with reality.
2) Can identify the continued partial or complete confusion and make arrangements for appropriate home care or placement.

Recommended References
"Breaking Through the Cobwebs of Confusion in the Elderly," by Carolyn Stevens. *Nursing 74*, August 1974:41–48.
"Caring for the Confused or Delirious Patient," by Gordon Trochman. *American Journal of Nursing*, September 1978:1495–1499.
"The Aged Patient: Chronic Organic Brain Syndrome." *NCP Guide #4:34*, Nurseco, 1978.
"The Aged Patient: Common Behaviors." *NCP Guide #2:26*, 2nd Ed., Nurseco, 1980.
"The Aged Patient: Reality Orientation." *NCP Guide #3:33*, Nurseco, 1977.
"The Aged Patient: Resocialization." *NCP Guide #3:34*, Nurseco, 1977.
"The Aged Patient: Transition to Communal Living." *NCP Guide #2:27*, 2nd Ed., Nurseco, 1980.
"The Confused Patient: Assessing Mental Status," by Marilyn Dodd. *American Journal of Nursing*, September 1978:1501–1503.
"The Confused Patient: Responses in Critical Care Units," by Margaret Adams et al. *American Journal of Nursing*, September 1978:1504–1512.
"The Confused Patient: Out of Touch with Reality," by Olive Wilkinson. *American Journal of Nursing*, September 1978:1492–1494.

The Patient Manifesting Denial

Definition: The manifestation of a person's inability or refusal to consciously acknowledge any thought, feeling, wish, or need of an external occurrence, or the threat of an occurrence.

LONG TERM GOAL: The patient will be able to interact with the environment in such a way that s/he maintains integrity and control but is not harmful to self.

General Considerations:

— **Denial occurs** as an unconscious effort to resolve emotional conflict and reduce the related anxiety. It occurs most often as a response to some threat to the status quo, i.e. trauma, illness, major life changes.
— **Nursing assessment** includes awareness of the manifestations of denial which include:
  — disbelief of diagnosis, symptoms, progress and/or information given;
  — changes information in such a way that it can be termed distorted;
  — refuses to discuss the hospitalization, surgery, trauma, or diagnosis;
  — refuses to participate in self care, either total body care or one aspect of care, i.e. colostomy care;
  — refuses medication, food, and/or all treatments;
  — refuses to follow recommendations such as bedrest, positioning, when these activities do not produce any increase in discomfort and may actually be more comfortable.
— **Nursing responsibilities** include monitoring activities of the patient so that the efforts at denial do not cause the patient harm, and supporting any patient efforts to understand what is happening to him.
— **Nursing interventions** should reflect the recognition of the patient's need to deal with the new situation at his own pace as long as this pace and method are not harmful.

Specific Considerations, Potential Patient Outcomes, and Nursing Actions:

1) Immediate Response to Recognition of Denial

The patient will eliminate the physically harmful aspects of the denial:
  — relieve anxiety through the establishment of a trusting relationship;
  — spend time with the pt., listen to him verbalize about areas of his life other than the focus of denial;
  — identify & support the pt. using other coping mechanisms, i.e. talking, crying;
  — attempt to identify the most threatening aspects of reality by observing when the pt. reacts the most intensely, i.e. pt. is on a thousand calorie diet & has the family bring in fattening food;

— do not support the denial but give pt. adequate care & converse with him frequently; do not avoid him;

— attempt to introduce realities slowly by beginning with the least threatening part of the reality, e.g. pt. refuses to begin looking at or caring for his colostomy; begin by discussing diet & then gradually move the conversation into discussing diet for colostomy pts.

2) Restoration to Adaptive Coping

The patient will accept the change and handle self care without supervision:

— continue to involve the pt. in own care by planning time, place & kind of care with him;

— praise & encourage any interest the pt. shows in knowing more about the change/illness;

— praise the pt.'s efforts in caring for self and/or beginning recognition of reality;

— help the pt. express angry and/or sad feelings by using open-ended questions, listening & spending time with him daily;

— spend time with significant others (SOs) to explain to them what is happening to the pt., and what they can do to assist & support the pt.'s positive efforts to cope;

— help other staff & SOs realize the importance of refraining from chastising the pt. &/or family when they are using denial to cope.

Discharge Planning and Teaching Objectives/Outcomes

1) (Patient/Family/Significant Other) Can discuss the positive and negative aspects of the change/illness.

2) Can follow those aspects of daily regimen that maintain life.

3) Can accept responsibility for possible effects of noncompliance with recommended regimen.

Recommended References

"Analogy: Weapon Against Denial," by Margaret S. Wacker. *American Journal of Nursing*, January 1974:71–73.

"Denial of Illness," by Sister M. Martha Kiening, in Carlson, Carolyn and Blackwell, Betty, *Behavioral Concepts and Nursing Interventions*, 2nd Ed., Philadelphia: J.B. Lippincott, Co., 1978:211–225.

"Mrs. Vinson Didn't Want Our Help," by Rhonda Lester. *Nursing 78*, August 1978:37–39.

"Solving the Riddle of Loss: 'Depression' and Other Responses." Filmstrips available from Nurseco, PO Box 145, Pacific Palisades, CA 90272.

The Patient Experiencing Dependency

Definition: A person's reliance on another person, persons, or things for continual support, reassurance and the meeting of needs.

LONG TERM GOAL: The patient will be interdependent, i.e. will rely on self and others.

General Considerations:
— **Dependency** is a passive means of control used to achieve one's desires for attention and input.
— **Confinement** in non-home like settings such as the hospital, extended care facility, etc., causes some dependency to occur and increases already existent dependency.
— **Nursing assessment** includes awareness of the manifestations of dependency which include:
  — refusal to participate in own care;
  — constantly asking staff to do for the patient what the patient is capable of doing for self;
  — asking staff to come into the room frequently;
  — constantly telling staff verbally and through behavior that s/he is "helpless" and unable to do anything alone;
  — refusal to learn new ways of caring for an altered self;
  — refusal and/or inability to make any decisions;
  — asking not to be transferred out of specialty units, eg. CCU, ICU.
— **Nursing responsibilities** include assessment of the patient's usual coping behaviors, and the length of time and extent of the dependency.

Specific Considerations, Potential Patient Outcomes, and Nursing Actions:
1) Immediate Response to Recognition of Dependency

The patient will perform at least one activity independently:
— attempt to identify the source of the dependency:
  a) ongoing lifelong style of coping; or
  b) environmentally stimulated: has the hospitalization decreased and/or removed so much of the pt.'s control that s/he has turned to dependency as a means of coping?
— do not criticize or openly acknowledge the dependent behavior;
— after careful explanation to the pt., set limits on the amount & type of dependent behavior that will be tolerated by the staff;
— give frequent, intermittent attention at times other than when the pt. asks for something;
— state when you will be back, return then or send someone else;

— praise any independent behaviors;
— explain to the pt. that you will not allow him to be so dependent, because you respect him & realize that he was able to do things for himself prior to hospitalization, & now you do not want to take this independence away.

2) Restoration to Adaptive Coping

The patient will identify needs which s/he can meet independently and needs with which s/he needs assistance:
— begin participation slowly & start with one activity only: eg., have the pt. wash own face, or hold something for you; praise efforts if s/he participates, but don't make an issue out of it;
— be supportive of & praise all independent efforts; if dependency is a lifelong pattern, you may not be able to change it but only set limits on the extent;
— plan the nursing care with the pt., have the pt. make some decisions, but start with one or two decisions, not all of them;
— give careful explanation about the pt.'s need to be more independent to family & significant others (SOs); tell them that they can be most helpful by getting the pt. to do some things for himself, & then praising these efforts;
— praise the efforts of the SOs when they assist the pt. to be independent.

Discharge Planning and Teaching Objectives/Outcomes
1) (Patient/Family/Significant Other) Can verbalize those areas where s/he can care for self and those areas where s/he needs assistance.
2) Can perform activities of daily living without constant attention.

Recommended References
"Caring for the Totally Dependent Patient." Nursing Grand Rounds. *Nursing 76*, July 1976:38–43.
"Giving the Patient an Active Role," by Tryon and Leonard in Skipper and Leonard, *Social Interaction and Patient Care*, Philadelphia: J.B. Lippincott, Co., 1965.
"Operant Conditioning in Chronic Illness," by Fowler et. al. *American Journal of Nursing*, June 1969:1226.
"Tad Appeared Helpless . . . Yet He Was Controlling Us," by Sherry L. Watkins. *Nursing 78*, June 1978:62–64.
"The Work of Getting Well," by Catherine Norris. *American Journal of Nursing*, October 1969:2118.

The Patient Experiencing Depression

Definition: An alteration in mood, usually related to a loss, and characterized by sadness, pessimism, despondence, hopelessness, and emptiness. It can also be aggression turned inward or the internalization of angry feelings.

LONG TERM GOAL: The patient will be able to talk positively and negatively about the loss, resume management of own life, and plan future goals.

General Considerations:
— **Depression is a response** to a real or perceived failure and/or a significant loss. See NCPG #1:31, "Responses to Loss." When resolution of the failure or loss is not complete, or complicated by additional failures or losses, the person will think that things cannot change and will "give up."
— **Nursing assessment** includes observing the patient for *behavioral manifestations of depression:* (1) stares off into space; (2) apathy (limited or no interest in self, others, or environment); (3) decreased initiative; (4) inability to concentrate; (5) decreased activity; (6) poor appetite; (7) complains of being, and looks, sad or tired all the time; (8) difficulty in getting to sleep at night and/or getting up in am; (9) feels sorry for self; (10) crying; and (11) withdrawal.
— **Nursing responsibilities** include an awareness of the difference between neurotic depression, described here, and psychotic depression (see NCP Guide #3:35, "The Patient Experiencing Depression (Psychiatric)"); an awareness of crisis intervention theory and practice, and an awareness of the signs and symptoms associated with suicidal risks. The focus of the nurse is on assisting the patient to regain control over own life and to express feelings s/he is experiencing.

Specific Considerations, Potential Patient Outcomes, and Nursing Actions:
1) Immediate Response to Recognition of Depression

The patient will verbally express feelings related to the painful event (i.e. failure and/or loss):
— make frequent, intermittent contact with the pt., both verbal & non-verbal;
— give attention consistently, even when the pt. is unwilling and/or unable to converse with you; this approach will establish you as an interested, caring person (depressed patients usually feel alone & worthless; a belief that someone is interested in & cares about them is the most helpful intervention);
— involve the pt. in self care & activities of daily living; start with one activity & gradually add others;
— suggest to the physician the use of anti-depressants, if you feel it is indicated;
— explore with pt. how s/he feels about listening to others' feelings (often people who have problems tolerating their own feelings tend to feel overwhelmed with others' feelings); practice sharing feelings of being overwhelmed & setting limits on listening to problems.

2) Restoration to Adaptive Coping

The patient will demonstrate the ability to carry out self care activities that are not physiologically impaired, make future plans and plan for discharge:

— continue to spend time with the pt. daily;
— use open-ended questions to elicit the pt.'s expression of feelings: e.g. "You look sad today. What is it that makes you feel this way?" acknowledge & reinforce any expression of feelings;
— do not tell the pt. s/he is not as sad or depressed as s/he feels; this approach only serves to reinforce the feeling that no one understands;
— make sure that everyone is aware of their responsibility for not chastizing the pt. when s/he is feeling sad;
— praise the pt. for any involvement in self care or other activities; encourage staff & significant others to praise pt. for these efforts;
— help pt. do things for self (many depressed pts. become dependent on others, but activity usually helps them to feel better);
— assist staff in their efforts to draw out the pt.; direct them to pay attention to him as much as possible;
— help pt. focus on meaning of loss, somatic symptoms, feelings tone: "You've had a hard time lately and you're learning to deal with your feelings." "You've lost functioning and you're going through grief and mourning."
— give positive reinforcement to reality & realistic expectations;
— identify problem areas & work out alternatives with pt.; take care to consider individual preferences & needs;
— assess areas in which pt. is making own decisions & give positive reinforcement to self-enhancing ones; assist with decision-making when profoundly depressed; as depression lifts, expect pt. to make own decisions with support.

Discharge Planning and Teaching Objectives/Outcomes

1) (Patient/Family/Significant Other) Can identify events/loss that led to feeling depressed.
2) Can recall the positive and negative aspects associated with the loss.
3) Can verbally express usual coping mechanisms for dealing with loss and how situational supports can assist to prevent depression.

Recommended References
"Dealing with Depression After Radical Surgery." *Nursing '79*, February 1979:47–49.
"Mr. Jarrett Was Ready to Give Up . . . but I Wasn't," by Diane Cole. *Nursing '78*, March 1978:40–41.
"Programmed Instruction: Helping Depressed Patients in General Nursing Practice." *American Journal of Nursing*, June, 1977:1007–1040.
"Responses to Loss: The Grief and Mourning Process." *NCP Guide #1:47*, 2nd Ed., Nurseco, 1980.
Suicide Assessment and Intervention, by Corrine Hatton et al. New York: Appleton-Century-Crofts, 1977.
"The Patient Experiencing Depression (Psychiatric)." *NCP Guide #3:35*, Nurseco, 1977.
"The Patient Who Is Suicidal." *NCP Guide #3:38*, Nurseco, 1977.

Dealing with Impending Death

Definition: The process or threat of loss of life.

LONG TERM GOAL: The patient will verbalize an understanding of what is occurring and how s/he is coping with it.

General Considerations:
— **Impending death** can occur as a response to traumatic events, short or long term illness. No matter the source, it causes the patient to bring forth whatever defenses s/he may have available.
— **Working through** the feelings and concerns associated with impending death involves five major stages, according to Kubler-Ross (see Recommended References). This is comparable to the three stages of the grief and mourning process as described in NCPG #1:31.
— **Lack of resolution** of any stage or completion of the total process may be related to the patient's fear of "acceptance" of death, and therefore loss of his ability to "hope" or desire to believe he will not die.
— **Nursing assessment** includes both physical and emotional needs of the patient: *physical needs*—explanations and information desired for decision making about ongoing medical treatment, level of treatment desired by the patient; pain tolerance and how the patient copes with pain, level of pain medication indicated and desired; nutritional preferences; cosmetic needs, including desire for wig, make up, prothesis; general comfort measures needed by the patient, e.g. frequent change of position, timing of procedures, interval of physical care; *emotional needs*—usual method of coping with threats and fears; desire for spiritual assistance; cultural and family practices desired by the patient; desire to talk about impending death with someone who will listen; patient and significant others' beliefs about patient's condition.
— **Nursing responsibilities** include a working knowledge of the grief and mourning process in order to make a nursing diagnosis, knowledge of resources available to the patient and his family, e.g. hospice care, thanotologists (a specialist in care of the dying), bereavement groups for the survivors. Interventions are directed toward comfort and supportive measures that assist the patient to cope *in his own way* with impending death. The only control the patient may feel s/he has at this time is control of how, when and with whom s/he dies. As much as is legally possible, do not take this control away from the patient.

Specific Considerations, Potential Patient Outcomes, and Nursing Actions:
1) Stage I: The patient will be able to use these coping mechanisms to begin to deal with his impending death:
   Denial and   — allow the pt. to utilize own method of coping as long as s/he is not physically destructive;
   Isolation   — know that pt. may have a feeling of "the need to protect others," to "fight the battle alone"; be available to spend at least 10 minutes with him daily either conversing or just being with him;
                  — assist the pt. to realize that denial and isolation are "normal" reactions to the news of the impending loss of life;

— answer questions about life, death & treatment honestly; the pt. doesn't want you to be harsh in your honesty, but s/he also doesn't want to be "fooled"; leave room in your answers for the pt. to maintain hope if s/he chooses to do so;
— do not reinforce pt.'s denial of his condition; when s/he makes an unrealistic statement ("I'm going to be back to work soon."), respond in a realistic manner, e.g. "It must be difficult for you right now."

2) Stage II: Anger   The patient will be able to express anger verbally about his impending death:
— allow & encourage the verbal expression of anger: remember, s/he is thinking, "Why does it have to be me?"; often this feeling is displaced on others; it is not personally directed at you but is a coping strategy that the pt. is using (see "The Patient Manifesting Anger," NCP Guide No. 1:21);
— know that the anger may be self-directed & associated with guilt about not seeking medical attention earlier; allow the pt. to express these concerns but not ruminate on them;
— allow open discussion of alternative treatment & life style options brought up by the pt.; assist him in consideration of these by giving clear, factual information about any alternatives; remember it is the pt.'s choice;
— listen to pt. express anger about distancing behavior from relatives & friends.

3) Stage III: Bargaining   The patient will be able to utilize this coping mechanism and associated behavior to try to prolong life;
— allow the pt. to cope by bargaining; s/he may use phrases such as "If only . . ." or "I could do . . .";
— ask the pt. about the importance of the events s/he is bargaining for; in this way, you express your availability to listen to him talk about his feelings;
— part of the bargaining may include the timing & interval of treatment or lack of such; allow the pt. the opportunity to make such decisions; be sure s/he is aware of the risks & consequences but allow him the decision.

4) Stage IV: Depression   The patient will verbally recognize the inevitable and allow himself to feel sad;
— know that the pt. may express the sadness verbally or by crying, silence, or talking; when pt. attempts to share sadness, do not try to cheer him up, but acknowledge his feelings;
— such questions as, "Am I going to die?" are a test of staff's willingness to listen to the pt. talk about his concerns, sadness & fears; respond, "Do you feel you are going to die?" then support & discuss responses;
— be aware that during this stage the pt. may be so overwhelmed with sadness that s/he no longer wants to talk or be involved in treatment; s/he may feel, "What difference does it make?"; focus on the normalcy of feeling sad & ascertain with him what difference coping with the impending death rather than giving up, will make to him;
— if pt. chooses not to move beyond this stage, feeling that if s/he stays depressed s/he does not have to make a decision about "fighting or accepting" death, gently remind him that staying depressed involves making a decision not to make another decision.

5) Stage V: The patient will accept the impending death as inevitable;
   Resolution
- acceptance involves the realization that death will occur & in preparation for such, the pt. has taken care of personal & family matters; is able to say death will occur & stops his struggle;
- know that often acceptance is not achieved but resignation is the method of resolution; resignation involves realizing that death will occur, but does not want it to happen, struggle continues & the pt. is not at peace with himself;
- spend time with pt.; encourage family & friends to continue to visit; the pt. does not want to be alone;
- the family may not be at the same level of coping as the pt.; share time with them discussing their feelings;
- allow the pt. control; encourage him to direct his care as much as possible; ask him what after death care he would like, i.e. spiritual care, funeral arrangements, family to be called.

Recommended References

"A Philosophy of Death Made Personal," by Sharon Hendrickson. *American Journal of Nursing*, January 1976:90.

"Dare to Care for the Dying," by Joy K. Ifemce. *American Journal of Nursing*, January 1976:88-90.

"Dealing Naturally with Dying," by Robert E. Kavanaugh. *Nursing '76*, October 1976:22-29.

"Experiences with Dying Patients." *American Journal of Nursing*—Feature Series, June 1973:1038.

"Hospice Home Care Program," by Barbara J. Ward. *Nursing Outlook*, October 1978:646-649.

On Death and Dying, by Elizabeth Kubler-Ross. New York: Macmillan Co., 1969.

"Surviving," by Patricia Chaney, Ed. *Nursing '76*, April 1976:41-50.

"The Advanced Cancer Patient: How He Will Live—And Die," by Ruth McCorkle. *Nursing '76*, October 1976:46-49.

"The Fine Example," by Dorothy W. Kimble. *Nursing '76*, July 1976:44.

"To Sharon with Love," by Maureen Cannon. *American Journal of Nursing*, April 1979:642-645.

The Patient Experiencing Fear

Definition: An emotional response to a consciously recognized internal and/or external source of danger.

LONG TERM GOAL: The patient will be able to interact with the environment in such a way that s/he recognizes factors and situations that cause him to be fearful.

General Considerations:

— **Fear** is a response that occurs in all individuals but can become especially acute in those with no previous hospitalization or with a previous traumatic experience. Fear may also present itself when a person associates his own anticipated experience with the traumatic experience of another, eg. family member, friend, job associate.

— **Nursing assessment** includes observing for behavioral manifestations of fear which include:
  - refusal of treatment;
  - putting on call light frequently;
  - making constant, unnecessary demands on staff;
  - constant attempts to please staff and do "what's right";
  - constant crying;
  - aggressive and/or critical with staff;
  - feeling a sinking sensation in stomach;
  - somatic complaints, such as nausea, diarrhea;
  - constant questioning about a care activity;
  - increased vital signs, perspiration.

  It also includes the assessment of the patient's response to the diagnosis, treatment and/or hospitalization in order to determine those activities or events which have caused the fear. It may be necessary to explore the intrapsychic meaning of the event(s) and relationship to a previous experience in order to determine the root of the fear.

— **Nursing responsibilities** include assessment and intervention which focuses on eliminating or reducing to a minimum the source of the fear, while enhancing the patient's control over other aspects of his care. Remember that loss of structure or loss of flexibility in daily living style can increase the intensity of the fear.

Specific Considerations, Potential Patient Outcomes, and Nursing Actions:

1) Immediate Response to Recognition of Fear

The patient will be able to identify the fear and its cause:
— attempt to identify the specific source of the fear;
— use indirect, open-ended questions such as, "What is it about being in the hospital that concerns you most?"
— give careful explanation of all that is to occur to the pt.; following explanations, have pt. tell you in his own words what you said & what it means to him; repeat this procedure as often as needed to ensure the pt.'s understanding;
— if you are unable to reduce the fear (eg. of dying during surgery) prior to the event, notify Dr. so appropriate corrective action can be taken; surgery may be cancelled.

2) Restoration to Adaptive Coping

The patient will be able to discuss his fears with others and accept treatment:
— spend at least 15 mins. with pt. each day; direct the conversation towards his responses to the hospital: "What thoughts are you having about the way your hospitalization is going?"
— listen to & positively reinforce the pt.'s attempt to talk about decisions that involve dangerous procedures or major life changes;
— do not make the decisions for the pt.;
— verbally & non-verbally assist the pt. in asking questions s/he may have about the progress and/or outcome of his diagnosis & treatment;
— direct questions about diagnosis & treatment not appropriate to nursing to the physician & explain the reason the pt. needs the answer, e.g. he is afraid of the outcome of his illness;
— involve & give explanation to other interested persons so they may reinforce the teaching you have done;
— allow friends & family to express their fears so they will be comfortable & supportive to the pt.; this intervention will be important in preventing the pt. from the realization of a fear of abandonment.

Discharge Planning and Teaching Objectives/Outcomes

1) (Patient/Family/Significant Other) Can verbally identify those aspects of own body and health care that cause fear.
2) Can utilize situational supports to reduce fear and accept treatment.
3) Can discuss information about developments in health care to prevent unwarranted fears.

Recommended References
"A Better Way to Calm the Patient Who Fears the Worst." *RN*. April 1977:46–33.
"Gaining Insight into Fear." *Nursing '78*, April 1978:46–51.
"Psychological Responses in Critical Care Units," by Margaret Adams et al. *American Journal of Nursing*, September 1978:1504–1512.
"The Frightened Patient," by Lisa Robinson. *Psychological Aspects of the Care of Hospitalized Patients*, 2nd ed., Philadelphia: F.A. Davis Co., 1972.

The Patient Manifesting Manipulation

Definition: The process of influencing another in such a way that one meets his own needs and wishes without regard to the needs, wishes, and functions of others.

LONG TERM GOAL: The patient will be able to express his needs and wishes in such a way that he demonstrates responsibility for his own actions and does not cause harm to others.

General Considerations:
— **Manipulation is a method** utilized by all persons to attempt to have the world come out as they want it. When manipulation is no longer seen as being acceptable because of the method or level, then it is perceived by others as negative and antisocial.
— Lifelong patterns of behavior are difficult to change and change only occurs if something else replaces the behavior; this new behavior must be perceived as rewarded and pleasurable.
— **Nursing assessment** includes a knowledge of the behavioral manifestations of manipulation which include: (1) pretends to be helpless; (2) pits staff, nurses, doctors against each other; (3) insincere complimenting of a staff member to her face, followed by negative comments about her to others; (4) makes undefined, ongoing demands; (5) makes excessive, unnecessary demands for staff time; (6) presents self as lonely and distraught in order to keep staff with him; this behavior continues to occur with no apparent resolution, even when intervention has occurred; (7) continues to act out (demand, yell, complain, etc.) even when repeatedly told that this is unacceptable behavior. Assessment also includes an awareness of the function and rewards of this behavior for the patient.
— **Nursing responsibilities** include reinforcing reality and preventing manipulation of self and others by the patient. Written, clear nursing care plans are the best tools to do this. Interventions should be based on principles of reinforcement theory.

Specific Considerations, Potential Patient Outcomes, and Nursing Actions:

1) Immediate Response to Recognition of Manipulation

The patient will verbally acknowledge that his present behavior is socially unacceptable and possibly physically harmful to himself and/or others:
— confront the pt. with his attempts at manipulation, then ignore manipulative behavior when possible;
— give praise, positive feedback & rewards such as social interaction, visitors, for non-manipulative behavior;
— allow the verbal expression of angry feelings;
— set limits on destructive behavior;
— tell the pt. to deal directly with you, otherwise you will continue to confront him with the efforts of manipulation;
— accurately record the instruction & information you give the pt. in the nursing notes & nursing care plans; this approach is useful in discouraging the pt. from changing, ignoring or distorting the communication;

— keep family informed of what you are doing & why.

2) Restoration to Adaptive Coping

The patient will accept responsibility for his actions, will be actively involved in his care and will accept the positive responses of others:
— plan nursing care plans & daily routine with pt.;
— decide who (pt. or nurse) is responsible for exactly what care, communicate this arrangement to staff, both verbally and in written plan;
— evaluate results of nursing care with the pt.;
— praise the pt.'s efforts in carrying out his responsibilities;
— accompany the Dr. on rounds to discourage the pt.'s distortion & misuse of what the Dr. has told him;
— clear, consistent communication among staff at all levels about the pt.'s manipulative behavior & the approach to be utilized is extremely important;
— praise staff & family members for their efforts at reducing the manipulative behavior of the pt.

Discharge Planning and Teaching Objectives/Outcomes
1) (Patient/Family/Significant Other) Can verbalize the way in which undesired manipulative behavior was being expressed.
2) Can accept the positive feedback for socially acceptable behavior.
3) Can ask directly for the needs to be met, questions answered.
4) Can wait for answers, needs to be met when the situation/need is not an emergency.

Recommended References
"Alienation" by Dorothy Block in Carlson, Carolyn and Blackwell, Betty, *Behavioral Concepts and Nursing Interventions*. Philadelphia: J.B. Lippincott Co., 1978:116–127.
"A Systematic Approach to the Evaluation of Interpersonal Relationships," by Linda Aiken and James Aiken. *American Journal of Nursing*, May 1973:863.
"Coping With a Seductive Patient." *Nursing '78*, July 1978:40–45.
"Debbie Got Attention the Hard Way," by Diana Guthrie. *Nursing '75*, November 1975:52–54.
"Mrs. Myers Played the Buzzer Game," by Joyce Kee. *Nursing '76*, July 1976:14–16.
"Two Types of Problem Patients . . . and How to Deal With Them," by Gertrude Ujhely. *Nursing '76*, July 1976:64–67.
"When It Comes to Difficult Patients, Mr. Billman Was a Showstopper," by Patricia Sharer. *Nursing '77*, September 1977:36–37.

The Patient Experiencing Pain

Definition: Pain is a situation that is the result of a single or class of stimuli; when perceived, it is accompanied by emotional and/or physical reactions.

LONG TERM GOAL: The patient will be free of pain and/or discomfort which impairs day to day functioning and the accomplishment of life goals.

General Considerations:
— **Pain** is the result of perception of noxious stimuli. The perception of pain is a protective mechanism and involves the nerve endings, spinal cord, brain stem, and cerebral cortex. The stimuli can be (1) *mechanical* (blow, friction), (2) *chemical* (microorganism, toxins, drugs), (3) *thermal* (hot and cold) or (4) *electrical current*.
— **Pain** can be (1) *superficial:* involves the cutaneous receptors, is localized, and has a sharp quality; (2) *deep:* from muscles, viscera; is more persistent, usually dull in nature and more diffuse; (3) *referred:* usually occurs at visceral level but actual point of focus of reaction or perception of pain is away from area of occurrence, eg. pain in an ischemic heart is felt in lower chest and/or left arm.
— **Pain threshold is based on several variables,** including: (1) type of pain stimuli, (2) location of pain stimuli, (3) cultural practices, (4) previous experience with pain in same or other body locations, (5) general body health and patient's perception of own health, (6) emotional health and fears associated with pain, and (7) source of pain: internal (body defense reaction) or external (clothing, dressings, position, noise).
— **Nursing assessment** includes observing for behavioral and physiological manifestations of pain which include: (1) pulse and blood pressure changes, (2) respiratory changes, (3) excessive perspiration, (4) nausea and vomiting, (5) changes in skin color, (6) generalized or localized muscle tension, (7) restlessness and tremor, (8) clenched fists, (9) spasm and muscle aches, (10) mood changes, (11) restlessness, (12) fear, (13) anxiety, (14) aggression, (15) impatience, (16) change in facial expression, (17) crying, groaning, grunting or gasping.
— **Nursing responsibilities** include knowledge of up-to-date treatment and prevention of pain, and an awareness of the fact that each individual has a different response to pain. *Intervention* should be directed toward relief of acute pain or treatment and reduction of chronic pain.

Specific Considerations, Potential Patient Outcomes, and Nursing Actions:

1) Immediate Response to Recognition of Pain

The patient will verbalize the feeling of reduction or alleviation of pain:
— determine the pt.'s pain history, previous responses as well as present ones;
— encourage the pt. to talk about his experiences with pain by showing interest in what he is saying, e.g. make eye contact, nod your head at times to respond to him, & especially, sit down with him when he is sharing feelings with you;
— utilize the knowledge you have about the pt.'s reaction & tolerance to pain as well as the doctor's orders to make your decisions about giving medication; do not withhold medication just because you feel the pt.'s pain is not real or should be adequately tolerated; remember . . . it is the pt. who is feeling the pain; there is suffering going on whether or not the pain exists or varies in level;
— when giving pain medication, tell the pt. about the medication & its expected effect; talk positively about it;
— utilize activities & conversation to help the pt. focus on something other than the pain; find out what s/he likes to talk about and/or activities s/he enjoys;
— do not reinforce the focus on pain in someone with chronic pain; instead, use behavior modification techniques & begin to reward non-pain focused behavior.

2) Restoration to Adaptive Coping

The patient will be able to distinguish between pain-related and non-pain-related activities; will engage in activities without constant thought of pain and will respond to reinforcement of non-pain-related living by making future life plans:
— plan with the pt. the kinds & timing of activities that can reduce, eliminate or minimize the suffering;
— pts. in pain cannot tolerate being rushed; when pt. is caring for self, allow as much time as s/he need to accomplish the task;
— allow the pt. to talk intermittently about the pain & suffering but not constantly; finding the cause of the suffering often relieves or reduces it;
— give positive feedback to the pt.'s efforts to share feelings & cope with the suffering;
— have friends, family, & staff available to pt. when s/he needs them;
— make sure all staff is aware of the pt.'s usual response to pain;
— hold pt. care conferences to discuss pt.'s responses to pain; plan approaches & write them in nursing care plan;
— take a few seconds & inwardly ask yourself, "What would I be like if I were suffering like this pt.?" Remember . . . identification of how we feel & respond increases our understanding of the variety of ways other people respond to situations, particularly painful experiences;
— facilitate significant others' understanding of the pt.'s suffering by giving careful explanations to them of how & why the pt. responds as s/he does;
— attempt to understand the religious, cultural & psychological influences in patterns of this particular pt.'s reaction to pain;

— teach pt. body relaxation techniques that can be utilized not only for pain reduction but during periods of tension & anxiety (these periods can elicit tension & anxiety in pain perception & reaction);
— teach pt. to use medication, support systems, diversional therapy & relaxation to cope with pain;
— for chronic pain, the patient should not only be aware of use of relaxation, behavioral & diversional therapy, but should have knowledge of outside resources such as pain clinics, reputable hypnotists & acupuncturists; refer PRN.

Discharge Planning and Teaching Objectives/Outcomes

1) (Patient/Family/Significant Other) Can verbalize events and conditions which influence the occurrence and level of pain.
2) Can identify medication use, diversional and relaxation activities that assist in the reduction or elimination of pain.
3) Can name community resources available for the ongoing treatment of intractable pain.
4) Can verbalize emotional responses to constant focusing on pain.

Recommended References

"Analgesics at the Bedside," by Nessa Coyle. *American Journal of Nursing*, September 1979:1554–1557.

"Angina: Teach Your Patients to Prevent Recurrent Attacks," by C. Walton and B. Hammond. *Nursing '78*, February 1978:32–38.

"Assessing Pain," by Ada Jacox. *American Journal of Nursing*, May 1979:895–900.

"Helping Patients Overcome the Disabling Effects of Chronic Pain," by J. Blair Pace. *Nursing '77*, July 1977:38–43.

"McGill-Melzack Pain Questionnaire," by Judith E. Meissner. *Nursing '80*, January 1980:50-51.

Nursing Management of the Patient with Pain, by M. McCaffery. Philadelphia: J.B. Lippincott Co., 1972.

"Pain and Suffering—A Special Supplement." *American Journal of Nursing*, March 1974:489.

"The Management of Pain: Using Analgesics Effectively," by M. DiBlasi and C. Washburn. *American Journal of Nursing*, January 1979:74–78.

"The Patient in Pain: New Concepts," by Jeanne Benoliel and Dorothy Crowley. *Nursing Digest*, Summer 1977:41–48.

Responses to Loss: The Grief and Mourning Process

Definitions: Loss—removal of something/someone of great value to the person.
Grief—the emotional responses that follow the perception, or anticipation, of a loss.
Mourning—the psychological processes that result following a loss.
Grief and Mourning Process—the process of coping with and adapting to the loss.

LONG TERM GOAL: The patient will be able to cope with the loss by completing each stage of the grief and mourning process.

General Considerations:
— There are **three categories of loss:**
  (1) sexual role identity, e.g. loss of family role, career role, sexual functioning, control over one's life;
  (2) self-image, e.g. loss of a leg, bowel functioning, self-respect;
  (3) nurturing, e.g. loss of a significant other.
  An actual or anticipated loss in any of these categories will trigger the grief and mourning process.
— The grief and mourning process involves **three stages,** according to Engel (see Recommended References): 1) shock and disbelief, 2) developing awareness of the loss, and 3) restitution.
— Each stage has its own **adaptive and maladaptive responses,** and time frame:
  (1) **Shock and disbelief:** Almost any behavior that helps the patient cope with the loss is *adaptive* for this stage. Common ones are denial, anger, crying, screaming; any kind of destructive behavior is *maladaptive*. This stage usually lasts *1-7 days;* after this time, the former adaptive behaviors may be considered maladaptive because the patient has not moved into the next stage.
  (2) **Developing awareness of the loss:** *Adaptive* behaviors are those which indicate beginning acknowledgement of the loss, e.g. "Maybe I will look OK with a prosthesis." "Do you think I'll be able to work with this?" Often the patient's behavior will swing "up" (as above) to "down" ("No, I'll never be able to cope with this."). Patients frequently blame themselves in this stage ("If only I had done . . ."). Any of the adaptive behaviors of stage one, as long as they are *interspersed* with this new behavior, are adaptive for this second stage. Destructive behavior is always maladaptive. This stage can last from *several weeks to months.*
  (3) **Restitution:** In this stage, the patient is able to recognize and deal with the loss, can put it aside and go on with the business of living. Typical behaviors include: making plans for the future; recalling comfortably and realistically both pleasures and disappointments associated with the loss. Full restitution may take up to *a year or more* and some people never complete this stage.
— **Nursing responsibilities** include an assessment of where the patient is in the grief and mourning process, his efforts to resolve the loss, and the results. Intervention should focus on helping the patient move along the continuum of the three stages of loss and provide resources for discharge planning.

Specific Considerations, Potential Patient Outcomes, and Nursing Actions:

1) Stage I:
   Shock and
   Disbelief

The patient will be able to use any non-destructive coping mechanisms to begin to deal with the loss;
— accept any behavior that is not physically destructive; do not try to cut it off or limit it;
— reinforce the occurrence of the loss while encouraging the pt. to talk about it; do not reinforce denial but rather, state, e.g., "It must be difficult to believe this is happening";
— spend at least 15 mins. each shift talking and/or just sitting & listening to the pt.; allow the pt. to direct the conversation;
— when appropriate, tell the pt. he is doing a good job of dealing with the loss;
— flex visiting hours for family/friends to stay PRN; try to fulfill any pt. requests.

2) Stage II:
   Developing
   Awareness of
   the Loss

The patient will be able to verbally express an awareness of the loss and its impact on him:
— incorporate a discussion of the loss in your daily conversations with the pt. and/or family; appropriate questions might be: a) "How do you see the effect of what has happened to you?" b) "How has your family coped with what has occurred?"
— when pt. begins to share sadness, encourage him to do so; sit & listen to what he says;
— reiterate that what he is experiencing is normal for his situation;
— involve the pt. in planning & doing some aspects of self care;
— restate questions the pt. has asked so that he can explore the answers with your assistance;
— make sure the pt. has ongoing situational supports to help him deal with the loss, e.g. friends, family, clergy.

3) State III:
   Restitution

The patient will be able to talk about the positive and negative aspects of the loss and make future goals:
— praise the pt.'s efforts to discuss the impact of the loss on his life; give positive reinforcement for future plans;
— allow the pt. control over as much of his care & method of resolving the loss as possible.

Discharge Planning and Teaching Objectives/Outcomes

1) (Patient/Family/Significant Other) Can express sadness over the loss but also plan for the future.
2) Can verbalize how he copes with losses and what situational supports are most effective.

Recommended References
"Grief and Grieving" by George Engel. *American Journal of Nursing*, September 1965:93.
"Planning For Retirement" by Elizabeth E. May. *Health Values: Achieving High Level Wellness*, May-June 1977:133–136.
"Sharing a Tragedy" by Judith Breuer. *American Journal of Nursing*, May 1976:758–759.
"Solving the Riddle of Loss: 'Depression' and Other Responses." Filmstrips available from NURSECO, PO Box 145, Pacific Palisades, CA 90272.
"Traumatic Blindness: A Flexible Approach for Helping a Blind Adolescent." *Nursing '79*, January 1979:36–41.
"Therapeutic Touch: Searching for Evidence of Physiological Change" by Dolores Krieger, Erick Peper and Sonia Ancoli. *American Journal of Nursing*, April 1979:660–662.
"The Grieving Patient and Family" by Mary Jo B. Marks. *American Journal of Nursing*, September 1976:1488–1491.

The Patient Experiencing Sensory Disturbances

Definition: A change in perception, level or type of response of an individual due to increased, decreased or absence of stimulation of the senses.

LONG TERM GOAL: The patient will regain and maintain sensory equilibrium.

General Considerations:
— **Sensory disturbances** occur in all acute care settings. With the advent of critical care units, life saving equipment, protective environments, and medical and nursing specialization, the intrusion on a person's environment, and/or lack of stimuli has increased and even contributed to morbidity rates.
— **Nursing assessment** focuses on observation of behavioral manifestations which include: (1) illusions, hallucinations and/or delusions, (2) withdrawal, (3) hostility (verbal attacks on staff), (4) crying or inappropriate affect, (5) confusion/disorientation of time, place, person, (6) sensory distortions e.g., incorrect perceptions of smell, touch, sight or response to treatment, (7) restlessness, (8) demand for constant reassurance about environment and treatment.
— **Nursing responsibilities** include an awareness of the *causes of sensory disturbances* to one or all senses (touch, smell, visualization and hearing). These causes include: (1) confinement in a small room; (2) lack of or excessive touching; (3) no verbal input or too much verbalization around the patient; (4) confinement in a windowless room; (5) discussion of hospital matters and/or information about other patients (these cause fear in addition to misperception of information related to the patient himself.); (6) continuous external stimuli, e.g., lights, monitors, staff/visitor verbalization; (7) lack of new stimuli; (8) placement in isolation; (9) change in external environment, e.g., new room, change in placement of equipment, personal supplies; (10) semi-consciousness and/or movement through different levels of consciousness causing a distortion (misperception) of what is heard, felt, seen or touched; and (11) separation from significant others. Interventions should focus on providing a stable environment for the patient by increasing or decreasing stimuli as needed.

Specific Considerations, Potential Patient Outcomes, and Nursing Actions:

1) Immediate Response to Recognition of Sensory Disturbance	The patient will be able to perceive and describe the components of his environment in an oriented, non-disturbed manner: — talk directly to the pt.; make eye contact; — use touch: give back rubs, massages, change position, stroke hair, etc.; — give the pt. frequent, intermittent attention; do not isolate the pt. physically or emotionally; speak to the pt. each time you enter or leave the room; — be aware of environmental monotony; use clocks, calendars, pictures, pt.'s personal possessions to stimulate & encourage pt. to explore his surroundings;

— give the pt. several periods of rest intermixed with stimulation throughout the day, rather than continuous stimulation;

— reduce or eliminate staff discussions of pts., hospital and/or personal matters in and around any pt.'s room or bed;

— identify what you are going to do each time you see the pt.; consider & utilize safety precautions as needed;

— some disturbances are caused by recumbent position alone; provide opportunities to sit, stand or be partially upright; give passive or active exercises;

— confusion that is physiological in nature cannot be controlled by behavioral approaches; however, it is important to approach the pt. often & give kind reassurances; do not increase fear & confusion by avoiding the pt.

2) Restoration to Adaptive Coping

The patient will be able to identify stimuli which are conducive to his treatment and recovery and stimuli which increase fear, anxiety, and restlessness:

— plan the care & daily activities with the pt.; evaluate the nursing care with the pt.;

— blind and/or deaf pts. have special needs due to the lack of these senses; make sure that these pts. have the opportunity to express these needs & have them met; communicate to all staff the sensory facilities the pt. may be lacking; e.g. blind, or without his glasses; deaf & without a hearing aid;

— ask the pt. to tell you when the stimuli is too little or too much . . . e.g., "It's so noisy." "I would like to rest." Attempt to reduce or increase the stimuli to meet the pt.'s needs;

— control levels of light, noise, odors, sights to tolerable levels; provide change of scenery, walks, rides, conversations with other pts., recreational or occupational therapy, & social activities as appropriate;

— have staff observe how the pt. is responding to them & the care they are giving (remember, the pt.'s response is a mirror of his need, not a response you take personally);

— make sure that all staff & significant others are aware of the pt.'s need for intermittent rest & stimulation; sensory overload mixed with deprivation does not allow the pt. to cope adequately with the hospitalization;

— provide the pt. with stimuli in the form of conversation, playing games, reading to him;

— refer pts. with long-term sensory impairments to the appropriate community resources, e.g. Society for the Blind.

Discharge Planning and Teaching Objectives/Outcomes

1) (Patient/Family/Significant Other) Can identify external environmental stimuli which are necessary for daily functioning.

2) Can identify external stimuli which cause fear, anxiety and reduce his ability to function.

3) Can identify and utilize sources of support to deal with sensory overload and/or deprivation situations.

Recommended References

"Bedrest and Sensory Disturbances," by Florence Downs. *American Journal of Nursing*, March 1974:434–438.

"Communication in the ICU: Therapeutic or Disturbing," by Mary Anne Noble. *Nursing Outlook*, March 1979:195–198.

"Sensory Alterations, Overload and Underload: Making a Nursing Diagnosis," by Mary Jane Barry, in M. Kennedy and G. Pfeifer, *Volume One: Current Practice in Nursing Care of the Adult—Issues and Concepts*. St. Louis: C.V. Mosby Co., 1979:33–45.

The Patient Experiencing Shock, Psychogenic

Definition: A state in which a person tries to insulate or protect self from a major event or imagined danger which is too much to handle all at once.

LONG TERM GOAL: The patient will be able to discuss the traumatic event and share positive and negative aspects of it.

General Considerations:
— **Psychogenic shock** is a response to a traumatic (real or imagined) event that confronts the individual. The person does not expect the event and cannot cope with the reality of it.
— **Nursing assessment** includes awareness of the manifestations of psychogenic shock which include:
  — silence;
  — crying;
  — denial of the causative event;
  — uncooperative manner;
  — unresponsiveness, appearing stunned or dazed;
  — apathetic, acting as if devoid of feeling;
  — unable to concentrate, to understand explanations and/or retain information;
  — feelings of helplessness, hopelessness or abandonment;
  — aimless wandering or puttering at small tasks;
  — hostility and/or blaming staff for the causative event.
— **Nursing responsibilities** include monitoring the patient's responses and activities since the patient is generally unable to cope without outside support.
— **Nursing interventions** should be directed toward allowing the patient time to come to grips with the situation and perceive the reality of it.

Specific Considerations, Potential Patient Outcomes, and Nursing Actions:
1) Immediate Response to Recognition of Psychogenic Shock

The patient will be able to allow others to assist him to cope:
— remain with the pt. for at least fifteen minutes or until replaced by another caring person;
— some denial of the event is important & necessary, but encourage the growing acceptance of reality;
— allow & encourage coping mechanisms such as crying, silence, walking, reliving the event;
— listen sympathetically, sharing the experience as the pt. permits you to do so.

2) Restoration to Adaptive Coping

The patient will return to responsiveness and responsible activity; will have a continuing human resource who will be helpful in a healthy way:

— assess what needs to be done & provide only the help that is really necessary;
— explore problem-solving options with the pt., but permit him to make his own decisions if they can be reality-based;
— allow the pt. to do as much as s/he can, but have another supportive person handle frustrating, complicated details & complex activities for the present;
— explain to the "supportive other" what the pt. is going through, how s/he is progressing, that the behavior is normal under the circumstances, & what can be expected of the pt. as s/he recovers from this state of shock (e.g. nightmares, possible physical complaints, resentment of others);
— verbally reward the "helper" for his interest, concern & willingness to be involved & available to the pt.;
— help this person to realize the pt.'s need to regain control of own life, to make decisions, & to do for self as much as possible;
— ask the "helping person" to use own personality strengths, i.e., warmth, humor, listening skill, etc., to sustain the pt. in moments of fleeting sadness, guilt, fear, etc.

Discharge Planning and Teaching Objectives/Outcomes

1) (Patient/Family/Significant Other) Can acknowledge the existence of the traumatic event.
2) Can allow others to be physically and emotionally supportive as needed.
3) Can demonstrate the ability to provide for own food, clothing and shelter.

Recommended References

"Grief and Grieving," by George Engel. *American Journal of Nursing*, September 1965:93.
"Helping Survivors Cope with the Shock of Sudden Death," by Patricia Sharer. *Nursing 79*, January 1979:20–23.
"Responses to Loss." *NCP Guide* #1:31, 2nd Ed., Nurseco, 1980.
"Sharing a Tragedy," by Judith Breuer. *American Journal of Nursing*, May 1976:758–759.
"Solving the Riddle of Loss:'Depression' and other Responses." Filmstrips available from Nurseco, PO Box 145, Pacific Palisades, CA 90272.
"The Simple Act of Touching," by James J. Lynch. *Nursing 78*, June 1978:32–36.

Chest Tubes & Bottles: Water-Seal Drainage

Purpose: To provide an outlet for trapped air and drainage to escape from the pleural cavity.

Nursing Responsibility: To keep chest tubes functioning properly so remaining lung tissue can re-expand.

General Principles:
— **Pressure inside the pleural cavity is negative;** atmospheric pressure is **positive.** If at all possible, the negative pressure will try to equalize by sucking in outside air; should this happen, the lung will collapse.
— **Underwater seal system:**
One end of the chest drainage tube will be in the patient's pleural cavity; the other end *must* be connected to a glass, or rigid plastic tube whose other end is *under water.* Otherwise, when the patient takes a breath, air will be drawn into the pleural cavity because of the pull of the negative pressure. As long as 3cm. of the tube is under water, and all connections are air tight, safety is ensured; as air and drainage come down the tube and into the water, they will be "trapped" there. The water level inside the glass tube will *fluctuate* with the patient's respirations, due to the pull of negative pressure. When the lung has re-expanded, this will cease.

Set-Up:
— A set-up will always contain one bottle but may contain two or three. Check out those available in your hospital, & which one is preferred by the surgeon; if disposable chest bottles are used, instructions are included with set-up.
— When the bottles are first set up, mark the original water level with tape or other indicator (so you will be able to measure the amount and rate of drainage).
— Secure chest tube to bed sheet with some slack between pin & insertion site to allow for patient movement & to prevent pulling on tube at chest entrance; be sure that no loop hangs below the level of the bed or interferes with patient movement.
— Slight suction is often applied to the bottles; check first with surgeon. If used, ensure that suction is kept at specified level *only.*

Maintenance:
— Make certain that all tubing is open and draining; check to see if water is fluctuating in the glass tube in drainage bottle.
— "Milk" the chest tube Q 15 mins. immediately after surgery until bleeding is stable or minimal, then at least BID & PRN. This will help push any clots and/or fibrin down the lumen, thus assuring patency.
— Check all connections for leaks; tape them securely PRN.
— Record amount of drainage QH times 8 hours, then Q4-8H PRN; know that sanguinous drainage of 40-60cc's (even 100cc's) in the first eight post-op hours is normal. If significantly more occurs, it may indicate hemorrhage.

Safety Precautions:

— Place bottles in a stand or other device to prevent them from being turned over, broken, etc.; ensure their protection during portable x-ray, visitors, etc.

— The tops of the bottles should be clamped or taped securely, with a warning written on them *not* to empty the bottles. Chest bottles should *never* be emptied unless specifically ordered by the surgeon.

— Keep at least one clamp, large enough to clamp chest tube, attached to patient's bed sheet (on same side as tube). If bottle should break, fall over, etc., clamp chest tube at once (to prevent air from being sucked into pleural cavity); notify surgeon immediately and get another drainage set-up.

— If necessary to move patient's bed, be sure chest bottles are kept *below* the level of the patient's chest. *Never* set bottles on the bed (or water may run into patient's pleural cavity).

— Patient may ambulate to bathroom or sit in chair while chest tube is still in place. if so, ensure *that under water seal is maintained*.

— Know, and share with patient, that chest tubes usually stay in place for 48 hours, and that s/he will have less discomfort in chest wall after they are removed.

Recommended References

"Discussion" in "Nursing Decisions," by Sarah Cook. *RN*, September 1978:90, 92, 94, 96.

Differentiating Hypoglycemia and Ketoacidosis (Hyperglycemia)

GOAL: The patient will recognize early symptoms of these two complications in order to prevent and quickly correct a potentially dangerous condition.

	HYPOGLYCEMIA (Insulin Reaction)	**KETOACIDOSIS** (Diabetic Coma)
Causes:	— too much insulin — not enough food (delayed or missed meals) — excessive exercise or work — diarrhea, vomiting, alcohol — sudden fear or anger	— too little insulin — too much or wrong kind of food — infection, illness, injuries, pregnancy — insufficient exercise — emotional stress
Onset:	— sudden (regular insulin) — gradual (modified insulin or oral hypoglycemic drugs)	— slow (days)
Symptoms:	(early) — hunger — sweating — pallor — cold skin — tremor — feeling of nervousness, anxiety — irritable behavior — decreased spontaneity — weakness, lethargy	(early) — thirst — increased urination (nocturia) — anorexia — nausea & vomiting — dim vision — headache
	(gradual) — blurred or double vision — mentally dull — change in behavior (negativistic, weepy, aggressive)	(gradually developing) — abdominal pain (cramps due to bloating from gastric atony) — constipation

---

- fatigue
- confusion, dizziness
- slurred speech
- slow, uncoordinated movement

Signs:
- shallow, rapid respiration
- rapid pulse
- dilated pupils
- tachycardia

- drowsiness
- headache
- weakness & fatigue
- listlessness

- flushed, dry skin (lack of skin turgor)
- fast, labored, deep breathing (air hunger)
- weak, rapid pulse
- subnormal temperature
- soft eyeballs
- acetone (fruity) breath odor
- hypotension
- coma

HYPOGLYCEMIA

Urine: — negative for sugar & acetone

Blood Glucose: — 60mg. or less/100 ml.

Treatment:
(1) give about 10 Gm. CHO:
- 4 oz. fruit juice, or
- 2 teaspoons cornsyrup, or
- 2 teaspoons honey, or
- 5 Life Savers, or
- 1 glass soft drink;
- if unable to swallow, squeeze concentrated glucose between gums & mouth (Reactose, Glutose, Cake Mate Decorating Jell);
- if necessary, IV Glucagon, 1 mg. may be given (can also be given IM or "subcu");

(2) obtain blood & urine specimens for lab testing;
(3) notify patient's doctor; (time of reaction, Sx & S, what given & response);
(4) give crackers and milk about one hour following initial treatment.

KETOACIDOSIS

— positive for sugar & acetone

— greater than 250 mg./100 ml.

(1) keep patient flat in bed and warm;
(2) if conscious, have patient drink sugar-free hot liquids such as coffee, tea, broth, bouillon;
(3) record intake & output;
(4) notify patient's doctor;
(5) obtain blood and urine specimens for lab testing;
(6) check & record vital signs & level of consciousness;
(7) prepare to administer parenteral fluids under a doctor's order;
(8) prepare to administer at least 20-40 units regular insulin with a doctor's order;
(9) connect to cardiac monitor & observe for potassium imbalance;
(10) refer to NCPG #2:48, "Potassium Imbalance," NCPG #3:40, "Acid-Base Balance," NCPG #3:48, 49 "Fluids & Electrolytes."

General Considerations:

— Oral hypoglycemics, while fraught with complications and now in disfavor, are still in use. Hypoglycemic attacks are more likely with age, renal and/or hepatic failure, alcohol ingestion, use of aspirin, phenylbutazone (Butazolidin) and the sulfonamides, Dicumarol and Chloromycetin.

— **Hyper**glycemia reactions **can** be a response to a previous **hypo**glycemic reaction, when the body tried to compensate for falling blood sugar levels by releasing glucose from liver. The amount of glucose released by the body and the CHO consumed by the patient often exceed what is needed and will produce elevated blood and urine sugar levels for about 24 hours (also known as Somogyi Effect). Treatment is to determine cause of **hypo**glycemia and correct it, **not** just to take more insulin for **hyper**glycemia.

Recommended References

"Acid-Base Balance." *NCP Guide* #3:40, Nurseco, 1977.

"Diabetic Ketoacidosis," by Mary Walesky. *American Journal of Nursing*, May 1978:872–874.

"Fluids & Electrolytes, Part A: Fluids and Part B: Electrolytes." *NCP Guide* #3:48, 49, Nurseco, 1977.

"Insulin Reactions vs. Ketoacidosis: Guidelines for Diagnosis and Intervention," by Norma Slater. *American Journal of Nursing*, May 1978:875–877.

"Potassium Imbalance." *NCP Guide* #2:48, 2nd Ed., Nurseco, 1980.

"Somogyi Effect: Managing Blood Glucose Rebound," by Joyce McCarthy. *Nursing 79*, February 1979:38–41.

General Dietary Principles for the Diabetic

LONG TERM GOAL: The patient will establish and maintain ideal body weight with proper nutrition.

Dietary Prescription:
- This represents the number of grams of carbohydrate, protein, and fat to be used in the daily food plan. It is calculated: *to provide an adequate intake* of vitamins and minerals; *to meet the caloric requirements* of the person, depending on the nutritional state, the normal daily activity needs and the ideal body weight as determined by sex, height, age, and bone structure; and *to satisfy special dietary considerations* for persons with health problems needing less fat, more protein or carbohydrate changes.
- To calculate the number of calories for a patient's diet, compute:
  - 20 calories per kg. ideal weight for losing weight;
  - 25 calories per kg. ideal weight for maintaining weight; or
  - 30 calories per kg. ideal weight for gaining weight or for increased activity needs.
- The well-balanced diet plan for most people provides food energy in the following proportions:
  - 20 to 25% protein (1 to 1.5 gr. per kg./body weight; more for children & adolescents);
  - 45 to 50% carbohydrates (about twice the amount of protein);
  - 25 to 30% fat (less than recommended in previous years).

Meal Planning:
Foods which have approximately the same amounts of carbohydrate, protein and fat have been grouped together in lists. Within a group, foods may be substituted for each other in the amounts given. Thus they are called **"exchange lists"** and were developed in cooperation by the American Diabetes Association, the American Dietetic Association and the Diabetes Section of the U.S. Public Health Service, Dept. of Health & Welfare. Copies of these lists, sample menus and special diet modifications (such as low sodium, bland or low fat) may be obtained from these sources as well as from Eli Lilly and Co.

General Rules (for all patients to know and follow carefully):
1) Eat all meals about the same time daily. Do not skip meals.
2) Eat only those foods, in the amount given, on the diet list.
3) Do not eat between meals UNLESS it is a part of your dietary plan, you are replacing food not eaten at a previous meal, or you feel an insulin reaction "coming on."

Foods Permitted As Desired:
- **Seasonings:** cinnamon, celery salt, garlic, lemon, mustard, mint, nutmeg, parsley, pepper, vinegar, vanilla, sugarless sweeteners.
- **Beverages:** coffee, tea, bouillon, fat-free broth, sugarless soft drinks.
- **Raw vegetables:** lettuce, endive, salad "greens," watercress, radishes, rhubarb, & dill pickles.

Foods to Avoid:
- Cake, candy, cookies, condensed milk, creamed foods, sugar, jam, jelly, preserves, marmalade, syrup, pies, and pastries.
- Alcoholic beverages, including beer and wine, unless special permission is obtained from physician and allowance is taken from dietary prescription.

Recommended References

Everything You Always Wanted to Know About Exchange Values for Food—But Were Unable to Find Out, by Marilyn Swanson and Pamela Cinnamon. Idaho Research Foundation, Inc., University of Idaho, Moscow, Idaho 1976.

Exchange Lists For Meal Planning and *A Cookbook for Diabetics.* American Diabetes Assn., 600 Fifth Ave., New York, NY 10020.

Sample Food Exchange Lists. Eli Lilly and Co., Indianapolis, IN 64206.

The Diabetics Cookbook, by Clarice B. Strachan. The Medical Arts Publishing Foundation, Houston, 1975.

Liquid Diet Substitutes for the Diabetic

Goal: The patient is able to meet daily dietary requirements in a liquid form whenever s/he is unable to chew, cannot take solid food, or has missed or failed to finish a complete meal.

Simplified Procedure (for temporary, occasional usage):

1) Weigh, measure or estimate as carefully as possible the amount of uneaten food in terms of carbohydrate, protein, and fat. Refer to exchange lists for help in estimating food values. For example: one ounce of meat, fish or cheese contains approximately 7 gm. of protein and 5 gm. of fat. One slice of bread or one-half cup of potatoes contains approximately 15 gm. carbohydrate and 2 gm. of protein.

2) Translate or convert the grams of carbohydrate, protein, and fat into a caloric equivalent. Remember that there are four calories in each gram of carbohydrate and protein and nine calories in each gram of fat.

3) Replace the missed calories with the appropriate amount of fruit juice using the list below:

Juice	Amount	Calories
Apple juice, canned	4 fluid ounces	64
Grape juice	4 fluid ounces	90
Grapefruit juice, canned, sweetened	4 fluid ounces	64
Grapefruit juice, canned unsweetened	4 fluid ounces	47
Orange juice, canned, sweetened	4 fluid ounces	65
Orange juice, canned, unsweetened	4 fluid ounces	56
Pineapple juice, canned	4 fluid ounces	60
Prune juice, canned	4 fluid ounces	84
Tomato juice, canned	4 fluid ounces	28

Standard Exchange List Procedure (for frequent, continuing meal replacement of more than one day's duration and for tube feedings as necessary):

1) List the total number of food exchanges allowed per day in each of the six categories (fruit, vegetable, meat, fat, bread and milk).

2) Substitute fruit juices for the fruit exchanges; puree and strain cooked vegetables and dilute with water for the vegetable exchanges; and select from the suggestions below for the meat, fat, bread and milk exchanges.

3) Distribute the liquid substitutes in balanced amounts every 1-2 hours throughout the waking day.

For 1 meat exchange and 1 milk exchange:	Eggnog made of 1 egg and whole milk, 8 oz., flavored with saccharine and vanilla.
For 1 bread exchange and ½ milk exchange:	Cooked cereal diluted with whole milk, 4 oz.
For 1 bread exchange and 2 fat exchanges:	Ice cream, ½ cup.
For 2 meat exchanges, 1 milk exchange and 1 fat exchange:	Mix 8 oz. of whole milk with 2 oz. melted cheddar cheese and 1 tsp. of margarine; flavor with celery salt.

Properties of Insulin Preparations

Type of Insulin	Activity and Time of Onset	Peak Activity and Time When Hypoglycemia Most Likely To Occur (with 7 a.m. admin.)
Regular, Crystalline	Short, 15-45 min.	2-4 hrs.; before lunch
Semilente	Short, 30-60 min.	4-6 hrs.; around noon
Globin	Medium, 2-3 hrs.	6-8 hrs.; afternoon
NPH	Medium, 1-2 hrs.	8-12 hrs.; afternoon to bedtime
Lente	Medium, 1-2 hrs.	8-12 hrs.; afternoon to bedtime
PZI	Long, 4-6 hrs.	14-20 hrs.; 9 pm to 4 am
Ultralente	Very slow, 5-8 hrs.	16-18 hrs.; 11 pm to 7 am

General Considerations:
— **Storage & Handling:** While insulin potency is ensured for longer periods of time when refrigerated, it is safe to store the vial(s) in usage at normal room temperatures of 60 to 80°. It will remain potent for 18-36 mos. Care should be taken not to freeze insulin or expose to temperatures above 95°F. to prevent loss of potency and clumping of suspended particles.
— **Administration:** For administration, insulin should **not** be cold as it stings, delays absorption, and may cause a local reaction. Insulin clings to glass and plastic over time & effective dosage administered will be significantly diminished; **so,** do **not** prepare insulin in syringe and store for later administration, and do **not** add insulin to IV containers of parenteral solution (give by IV push method, close to insertion site).
— Insulin in **U-100** vials is rapidly becoming the standard for use. It is believed to be more purified, with fewer contaminants, thereby causing fewer untoward reactions. Because it eliminates dual calibration syringe confusion (of U-40 & U-80 types), administration without error is more likely to occur.
— For patients with visual difficulties, a preset attachment is available for syringes, which limits the amount withdrawn to a predetermined amount.
— Modified insulins settle upon standing and should be rotated gently to redistribute the contents. The bottle should never be shaken because air bubbles in the solution make accurate withdrawal especially difficult.

- Some syringes with removable needles have as much as 0.1cc "dead space" (insulin left in needle & hub after injection is given) which may result in an insulin dosage error of up to 10 units (U-100 insulin). To correct for this, either withdraw different types of insulin in separate syringes for separate injections, or else use syringes with the least amount of dead space and allow for it accordingly.
- To prevent skin reactions, all injections of insulin should be made with a sharp pointed ⅝ in. needle inserted at a 90° angle (perpendicular) to the stretched skin. Lift a skin fold for especially thin persons, so that the insulin goes into the subcutaneous tissue, below fat and outside muscle. Overweight persons should use longer needles of 1-1½ in. length, as needed. Always aspirate to be certain that needle is not in a blood vessel.
- Use a written chart of systematic rotation of injection sites, to avoid usage of the same general area oftener than two to four weeks. Whenever possible, the patient's family or friends should be enlisted to give injections so the patient's buttocks, both upper arms and back can be used. In this way the original site may not be re-used for as long as six weeks, thus reducing chances of lipodystrophy and absorption problems. Instruct patient to avoid injections near joints, body folds, scar tissue, moles, cuts or inflamed areas.
- **Absorption:** Know that the times listed on charts for onset, peak, duration of action are for "average" person's response; patients may respond differently based on vascularity and absorption of injection site as well as physiological body variations, hormone levels and antibodies to insulin. Changes in insulin dosage will be made according to individual patient's response, lifestyle, exercise level, diet, stress, and job requirements.
- **Skin reactions:** May be (a) local, temporary indurations or wheals that last a week or several months; (b) atrophy: simple dimpling or extensive pitting of subcutaneous tissue; and (c) hypertrophy: spongy, swollen mass of scar tissue. Atrophy is more common in women, hypertrophy is more common in males and both kinds are common in children, more than adults. An effective rotation plan can diminish disfigurement. Use of purified, single peak insulins also cause fewer reactions.

Recommended References
How To Take Insulin. Monoject, 1831 Olive St., St. Louis, MO 63103 (available in French or Spanish), 1977.
"Insulin: Paving the Way to a New Life," by Lawrence Wolfe. *Nursing 77*, November 1977:38–41.
"Preventing Insulin-Induced Lipodystrophies," by Dorette S. Welk, RN, MS. *Nursing 79*, December 1979:42–45.
"Teaching Patients to Rotate Injection Sites," by Ann McClung Fonville. *American Journal of Nursing*, May 1978:880–883.

Recommended Care of the Feet for Diabetics
(and Other Patients with Poor Circulation)

LONG TERM GOAL: The patient has adequate circulation to extremities; the patient is free of infection and protects feet from injuries; the patient demonstrates the ability to give own proper foot care or is able to seek necessary assistance.

General Considerations:
— **Peripheral neuropathy** is one of the most common complications of diabetes. Diminished sensation as well as vascular insufficiency contribute to infection and slow healing of injuries.

— Proper care of the feet can prevent most serious foot problems; saving the lower extremities from amputation is a prime objective. Nurses should teach and supervise patients (or a helping family member or friend) how to take good care of their feet. They should refer to a podiatrist those with special needs.

— **Walking** daily is very effective for improving circulation and healing minor ulcers or infections. Antibiotics, debridement and warm, moist soaks may also be ordered PRN. Patients should also be encouraged to refrain from using tobacco in any form.

General Principles of Proper Foot Care:
1) Wash feet daily in warm water and mild soap. Rinse well and dry gently but thoroughly with a clean, soft towel.
2) Apply lanolin, cocoa butter or lotion to dry areas. Sprinkle powder between toes to combat moistness. Separate overlapping toes with lambswool.
3) Exercise feet at least three times daily by: walking; bending feet up, down, sideways, and in circles; curling and stretching toes.
4) Cut toenails straight across, even with the end of the toe. Be careful not to cut too short or to cut skin. Use an emery board to smooth edges and avoid tears. Clean under nails with an orangewood stick, gently and cautiously.
5) Have a podiatrist remove corns, calluses and trim nails that require special attention (e.g. thickened, ingrown) or for the visually handicapped person.
6) Inspect feet daily for redness, cracking, blisters, ulcers, swelling, infection, or changes in color or appearance. Report any of these signs promptly to doctor.
7) Wear clean, colorfast, cotton socks (white often preferable) and be certain they are not tight fitting. Choose properly fitting leather shoes and hard-soled, supportive houseslippers. Inspect for nail points, rough stitching areas or other lumps that may cause irritation. Avoid vinyl or rubber shoes which do not allow feet to breathe. Break in new shoes gradually for short periods. Alternate pairs of shoes to allow them to air out and regain shape. Wear socks to absorb perspiration, even with tennis shoes and houseslippers. Avoid, as much as possible, thongs, sandals, open-toed or open-heeled shoes. Do not go barefoot, even on beach or swimming pool decks.

8) Avoid girdles, garters, knee high stockings or tight belts which interfere with venous return. Avoid sitting with crossed legs. Do not stand for long periods. Elevate feet when resting.

9) Since sensory reactions are diminished as age and disease progresses, avoid hot water bottles, heating pads, excessively hot water, sunburn, excessive cold. Wear bed socks if needed to keep feet warm. Do not use strong antiseptics or linaments.

10) Report promptly to doctor first signs of infection, discoloration or drainage, athlete's foot and fungus nail infections (yellow, thickened nails). For first aid of minor injuries, cleanse promptly, apply alcohol and a dry, sterile dressing. Use no medicated liquids or ointments without doctor's approval.

Recommended References

"Diabetic Peripheral Neuropathy," by Joan Petrlik. *American Journal of Nursing*, November 1976:1794–1797.

"Foot Care for Diabetics," by Emma Ventura. *American Journal of Nursing*, May 1978:886–888.

The Effects of Hospitalization, Part A: Tension-Producing Causes

Definition: Hospitalization is the confinement of a person in a setting designed to diagnose, treat or monitor physiological and/or psychological disturbances.

LONG TERM GOAL: The patient will demonstrate ability to participate in his care, make adaptive decisions regarding treatment and care, act interdependently with the health team, and express feelings of sadness over the loss of normal functioning.

General Considerations:
— **Hospitalization** is accepted as a means of treating problems that cannot be handled on an out-patient basis. The level of manifestation of behavioral responses to the dependency caused by hospitalization is a direct result of the intensity of loss of control experienced by the patient.
— **The stress of hospitalization** may intensify symptoms and increase the length of time required for coping.
— **Nursing responsibilities** include assessment of the patient's behaviors, need for situational supports, and the impact of hospitalization on his on-going life style.

Specific Considerations: Common Feelings of Patients that Produce Tension:
1) A Feeling of Powerlessness
Definition: The feeling of the ordinary individual that s/he cannot influence or understand the very events upon which his life and happiness are known to depend. The person feels that s/he has no power to control what is happening.

Some Causes: — Exposure to an artificial, temporary, governing body, such as the hospital staff;
— threat of force, such as, "If you don't eat, we will start an IV.";
— threat of punishment for not abiding by the rules, that is, rejection or avoidance by nursing staff, failure or delay in answering call bells, etc.;
— fear of the unknown (someone walks into the room; although the patient knows him, s/he doesn't know what is going to happen);
— imposed restrictions and limitations, e.g. best rest, no BRP, need for help with ADL.

2) A Feeling of Isolation
Definition: The condition or situation of being set apart from others.
Some Causes: — Physical separations from others for a long period of time with no interaction;

— emotional separation from others through use of another language or by treating the patient as if s/he were an object upon which certain tasks are to be performed (e.g. viewing patient as a diagnosis, rather than an individual, equal, client, or health consumer);

— separation from family and friends.

3) A Feeling of Loss

Definition: A state of being deprived of or of being without something one has previously had.

Some Causes: — Real or anticipated loss of a body part or functioning of a body part;

— real or anticipated loss or change in a person's own view of self (self-image);

— loss of a loved one;

— loss of control over self, others, or the environment.

4) A Feeling of Culture Shock

Definition: The response that occurs whenever an individual is placed in an unfamiliar situation in which his known ways of dealing with the situation are ineffective and in which adaptation clues are absent.

Some Causes: — Moving a person from a known to an unknown environment;

— exposure to a new language, e.g. hospital jargon, medical terms;

— exposure to a new authority structure;

— enforced dependency and submissiveness.

Discharge Planning and Teaching Objectives/Outcomes

1) (Patient/Family/Significant Other) Can verbally express behavioral manifestations used as a means to cope with hospitalization.

2) Can verbally express those areas of care where s/he wants to be independent and those areas where s/he is willing to be dependent.

Proceed to NCP Guide No. 1:41: Effects of Hospitalization, Part B: Assessment

Recommended References

"Familiarity: Therapeutic? Harmful? When?," by Seymour Shubin. *Nursing '76*, November 1976:18–21.

"From Model Patient to Little Tyrant," by Carol Wiedner. *Nursing '78*, April 1978:36–39.

"How Well Do Patients Understand Hospital Jargon," by Bonnie Casper. *American Journal of Nursing*, December 1977:1932–1934.

"Jack Wanted to Direct His Care His Way," by June Ludwig. *Nursing '75*, August 1975:10.

"Ordeal," by Patricia Chaney, Ed. *Nursing '75*, June 1975:27–40. June 1975:27–40.

"Responses to Loss: The Grief and Mourning Process," *NCP Guide* #1:31, 2nd Ed., Nurseco, 1980.

"The Patient's Bill of Rights: A Significant Aspect of the Consumer Revolution," by Quinn and Somers. *Nursing Outlook*, April 1974:240.

"Why Did Mr. Howard Stop Singing for Us?" by Nancy L. Bradfield. *Nursing '78*, November 1978:46–48.

The Effects of Hospitalization, Part B: Assessment

Goal: The patient will use adaptive coping mechanisms that enhance treatment and encourage rapid recovery.

General Considerations:
— **Assessment** is the collection and evaluation of data gathered about the health status of the patient. This data is gathered from a variety of sources including the patient interview. It is utilized to make a nursing diagnosis and plan nursing interventions. (See NCPG #1:46, "Restoring +: An Assessment Tool.")
— **Nursing responsibilities** include the assessment of the patient's **response** to hospitalization, along with physiological and psychosocial data regarding the reason for hospitalization.

Specific Considerations:
1) **Assessment includes** obtaining answers to these questions:
   1.1 What is the patient's usual way of living, loving and coping? (Both past and present ways).
   1.2 What are the patient's past and present experiences that have had a significant influence on him? (e.g. orphan, recent death of loved one).
   1.3 What is the patient's basic personality? (i.e. introverted or extroverted, dependent or independent, pessimistic or optimistic?)
   1.4 What is the patient's knowledge of and beliefs about medical concepts, medicine and medical practice?
   1.5 What are the patient's religious beliefs and how do these influence his responses to illness and medical treatment?
   1.6 What is the reason for the patient's hospitalization?
       a. As stated by the patient?
       b. As related by others: family, doctor, hospital staff?
   1.7 What are the patient's expectations with regard to:
       a. Course of illness or disability?
       b. Outcome of the hospitalization?
       c. Medical treatment s/he will receive?
       d. Care to be provided by the nursing staff?
       e. His family's involvement in his care and treatment, and emotional support?
   1.8 What influence did the patient's method of admission to the hospital have? For example, a) was s/he admitted through the emergency room, admitting office, or the outpatient department? Under own power or brought in by others? b) Did s/he have to wait a long time before getting to his room? c) Was there any contact between the patient and the hospital staff during the waiting period? d) What is the patient's

perception of the kind of contacts he has had during and since admission?

1.9 What is the patient's initial reaction to the staff on the unit? Is s/he talkative? Withdrawn? Quiet? Asking questions? Hostile? Especially accommodating, cooperative, or submissive?

Taking the data gathered from these questions, plus the data on the Restoring + Assessment form, you are now ready to formulate and write out the Nursing Care Plan (See NCPG #1:48).

2) **Writing out the Nursing Care Plan:**

 ⁻ Making a Nursing Diagnosis is the next step. Validate your perceptions with the patient, set goals together. For information on specific behavior problems, refer to section B, "Patient Behaviors," NCPG #s 1:20–33.

Recommended References

"Communication Blocks Revisited," by Sister Mary James Ramaehers. *American Journal of Nursing*, June 1979:1079–1080.

"Elements of a Psychological Assessment," by Joyce Snyder and Margo Wilson. *American Journal of Nursing*, February 1977:235–239.

"Helping Your Patient Sleep: Planning Instead of Pills," by Gina P. Zelechowski. *Nursing '77*, May 1977:62–65.

"Nursing Assessment Form: Restoring +." *NCP Guide* #1:46, 2nd Ed., Nurseco, 1980.

"Patient Behaviors." *NCP Guides* #'s 1:20-33, 2nd Ed., Nurseco, 1980.

"Patient Needs on Admission" by Anne Porter et al. *American Journal of Nursing*, January 1977:112–113.

"Problem Patients Do Not Exist," by Jean Scheideman. *American Journal of Nursing*, June 1979:1082–1083.

"Steps in Writing Nursing Care Plans." *NCP Guide* #1:48, 2nd Ed., Nurseco, 1980.

"Trivia, Illusions, and Quirks. What They Can Tell About Your Patients," by Sandra R. Stafford. *Nursing '75*, September 1975:6–7.

"When Your Feelings Get in the Way," by Lynne B. Jungman. *American Journal of Nursing*, June 1979:1074–1075.

The Effects of Hospitalization, Part C: Prolonged Confinement

Definition: The confinement of an individual in an institutional setting for a prolonged period of time (two weeks or longer). This prolonged confinement may produce behavioral changes not seen in the early part of the confinement.

LONG TERM GOAL: The patient will be able to verbally express a description of his method of coping with prolonged confinement and self-care activities which make him feel most in control of his life.

General Considerations:

— **Prolonged confinement** results in behavioral changes not seen previously because the patient has not expected to give up control for this length of time. Generally the patient is willing to abide by the "rules of others" when the time frame is short or when s/he expects and prepares for a major change of control. When prolonged confinement occurs in unexpected situations, the patient must deal with additional stress and loss.

— **Nursing responsibilities** include the awareness of possible causes of the behavioral changes which include:

(1) basic personality needs not being met, e.g.: an independent person is forced to be dependent over a period of time;

(2) fear of coping again in an environment other than the hospital;

(3) fear of death;

(4) sensory disturbances (see NCPG #1:32);

(5) deprivation of affection;

(6) sexual abstinence.

— **Nursing assessment** includes awareness of the common behavioral manifestations which are a response to the confinement. These include:

(1) a talkative patient becomes withdrawn, no longer interacts with staff and/or family;

(2) a patient who has been actively involved in his care begins to refuse to participate and/or makes excuses consistently for not participating; in his care;

(3) a patient who has been open with the staff withdraws and becomes passive-aggressive, that is, instead of asking for things or needs openly, as before, the patient begins to intermix complaints and hostility with being nice and saying all is fine;

(4) a patient becomes confused and disoriented with no apparent physical cause for the change;

(5) definite personality changes, e.g. an optimist becomes a pessimist; an independent patient becomes overly dependent.

— **Nursing interventions** include an awareness of the patient's need for ongoing control, encouragement and praise of those areas the patient can control, as well as the following approaches:
   (1) converse daily with the patient; incorporate these items into the conversation:
      a. What is the person's level of awareness of changes in himself?
      b. What recent losses or significant changes have occurred?
      c. How does the person see these changes in relation to his usual ways of coping?
      d. What does the patient want the staff to do to assist him to cope with these changes:
         — provide more time for visitors?
         — provide more reading material?
         — read to him?
         — provide weekend furloughs?
         — provide games and someone to play them with him?
         — provide written information about the patient's illness? e.g. booklets, American Cancer Society, etc.
         — provide a roommate who is conducive to sharing time and interest with him?
   (2) Point out the real and identified changes in behavior to the patient; the patient may not realize these changes have occurred. (e.g. "I notice you are angrier lately. Would you like to talk about it, about what may have produced the change?")
   (3) Provide information to the staff on how the patient has changed; encourage staff to be aware of the patient's attitude about how s/he will cope.
   (4) It is important to spend some time each day with the patient; this time should be directed towards activity and/or conversation but it must incorporate a willingness to be involved in the patient's efforts to cope with these changes.
   (5) Fear and feelings associated with a loss or threat of a loss may be playing an important part in the patient's response. An understanding of the concepts of loss and fear is necessary for effective intervention (see NCP Guide No. 1:28, "Fear" and NCP Guide No. 1:31 "Responses to Loss").

Discharge Planning and Teaching Objectives/Outcomes

1) (Patient/Family/Significant Other) Can identify behavioral changes related to prolonged confinement, and ways s/he coped with them.
2) Can utilize situational supports to adapt to continued confinement or readjustment to home environment.

Recommended References

"Instilling Hope," by Barbara J. Limandri and Diana W. Bagle. *American Journal of Nursing*, January 1978:78–79.
"Providing Motivation," by Adaline B. Chamberlin. *American Journal of Nursing*, January 1978:80.
"Survivors of Serious Illness," by Dorothy W. Smith. *American Journal of Nursing*, March 1979:440–443.
"The Seminar on the Chronically Ill," by Rev. David C. Duncombe. *Nursing Digest*, September-October 1975:22–25.

Basic Principles for Changing a Temporary or Permanent Appliance
(for the Patient with an Ileostomy or Urinary Stoma)

GOAL: The patient will have a securely fitting ostomy appliance without leakage, skin irritation or discomfort.

General Considerations:
— Teach the patient the entire procedure, step-by-step as given below or as modified by the type of appliance or commercial preparations preferred. Post this guide or a re-copy with modifications at the patient's bedside. Let the patient take this copy home with him.
— Provide the patient with at least three weeks' supplies for changing appliance and the name and address of a local supplier of ostomy products. After the patient is comfortable with the procedure and the basic principles, encourage him to experiment with products and appliances until s/he finds what works best. Joining a group of ostomates is one of the best ways to learn of new products or better ways of managing one's own ostomy.

Basic Principles:
1) **Provide** for sufficient light, working space and privacy so that nurse and patient can work together comfortably. Explain each step and its purpose to the patient.
2) **Arrange all necessary equipment** in readily accessible positions to save time and energy. Efficiency helps maintain the patient's confidence in the nurse's competence. Suggested items include:
   — basin for emptying ileostomy pouch;
   — graduated pitcher for measuring amount of fecal discharge;
   — asepto syringe for rinsing one-piece pouches;
   — eye dropper for applying solvent;
   — solvent to remove cement or adhesive from skin and appliance (faceplate type); acetone or special non-irritating solvent is preferable (Take precautions to prevent spillage and to prohibit smoking in the area.);
   — manicure scissors for easily cutting hole in some types of appliances;
   — basin of warm, not hot, water for rinsing skin and appliance;
   — cotton balls (or gauze pads) and applicator swabs for cleansing skin and applying skin protectives;
   — facial tissues to make a stoma collar for preventing ileostomy leakage upon surrounding skin;
   — thick, wide rubber bands, or suitable clamps, for affixing pouch to face-plate or for closing drainage hole in one-piece plastic bags;
   — *plain*, not compound-type, tincture of benzoin for skin protection (toughens and heals); compound-type benzoin should *not* be used, because it has been found to contain skin-irritating impurities;

— karaya gum powder (in sifter can or spray bottle) or commercially prepared karaya gel wafers or rings;

— aluminum hydroxide gel, or other antacid preparation, to mix with karaya powder for peristomal skin protection and healing;

— Stomahesive (R) or Davol Reliaseal (TM) for adhesive properties on weeping, irritated skin;

— commercial ostomy cement;

— deodorant for placing in bag and rinse water;

— room deodorant;

— substitute belt if needed;

— temporary or permanent appliance for use while present one is discarded or cleaned, dried and aired;

— foam discs to use between faceplate and skin, if desirable, to assure patient comfort; these must be non-porous foam rubber or neoprene pads, not sponge, to retard leakage;

— talcum powder to sprinkle between collection pouch part of bag and skin for absorbing perspiration and diminishing irritation; a cotton handkerchief can also be placed here for absorption and comfort;

— stoma-measuring gauge or template; stoma shrinks during the first eight weeks; to prevent skin excoriation from drainage, it is necessary to measure stoma each time and fit appliance snugly;

— pencil to trace stoma size hole (plus $\frac{1}{16}$ to $\frac{1}{8}$ inch clearance) on waxed sheet covering adhesive and foam discs;

— small, hand mirror so patient can see procedure better.

3) If **temporary one-piece postoperative appliance** is neither loose, nor leaking, **simply empty bag** by snipping hole in one lower corner and collect drainage in a basin. Measure and record amount, color, consistency. Rinse inside of pouch by squirting clear water with an asepto syringe. Wipe bag gently with tissue, taking care to support its attachment to the skin. Wipe away fecal discharge with damp gauze. Apply paste-like mixture of karaya powder and antacid solution around stoma at the muco-cutaneous junction (working through the hole you've cut in the bottom of the bag, of course). Straighten sides of bag, express air, and close opening tightly with a rubber band or suitable clamp.

4) **To remove a one or two piece appliance from skin,** drip solvent slowly between edges of appliance and skin. Gently and carefully pull appliance free using additional solvent if necessary. Since solvents are powerful de-fatting agents, they should be promptly cleansed from skin with water, not soap. Rinse thoroughly and pat dry, completely. Remove excess cement from faceplate of permanent appliance to prevent build-up and odor.·

5) **Measure stoma diameter** with ruler or template gauge, adding $\frac{1}{16}$ to $\frac{1}{8}$ inch clearance.

6) **Swab skin** with plain tincture of benzoin to one-half inch beyond radius of appliance; allow to dry. Apply second coat covering area around stoma completely up to muco-cutaneous junction. Some use spray Skin Prep (R) or similar product.

7) **Fold facial tissue** in thirds lengthwise and wrap a collar of tissue around stoma. It may be necessary for patient to hold this in place. For a large, active stoma, a cheesecloth gauze fluffed inside collar provides additional absorption to prevent leakage on skin.

8) **Draw correct size circle** on protective waxed sheet or film over adhesive disc, foam disc, or adhesive side of one-piece polyethylene appliance. Cut hole with a smooth edge.

9) **Apply a mixture** of karaya gum powder and antacid solution to skin around stoma. At least two coats are needed for adequate protection. This is also good to fill uneven skin depressions around stoma. Instead of the karaya-antacid mixture, a commercial karaya gel ring/wafer or a karaya seal type bag may be used. Squibb Stomahesive (R) or Davol Reliaseal (TM) skin protection barrier, adhesive wafer may also be used, especially if the skin is excoriated, weeping or irritated. In either case, karaya rings or adhesive wafers must leave *NO* margin of exposed skin around stoma to break down with ileal drainage.

10) **Apply cement** in small drops and spread with fingers or brush to make a thin coat over entire faceplate (or skin side) of appliance. Applying surgical cement to adhesive-backed one-piece appliances enhances adherence and insures longer wearing times. Allow to dry completely and apply a second coat of cement. Drying takes at least two to five minutes (longer in humid climates). While waiting, apply two coats of cement to skin, being certain that cement is dry to a light touch of finger before applying a second coat. Trapped moist cement produces irritation. For time-saving convenience, double-backed adhesive sheets (mentioned above) are recommended, although more expensive. They are recommended for excoriated skin because they contain wet adhesives as well as dry adhesives to adapt to the different conditions of the irritated skin.

11) **Remove tissue collar** and gauze over stoma.

12) **Apply faceplate** (with attached foam disc, if used), centering hole around stoma with even margin all around; seal by pressing smoothly with fingers from inner to outer edges, preventing wrinkles.

13) **Put deodorant** preparation into pouch. While patient or assistant steadies the faceplate, attach the pouch to the faceplate. Some appliances have their own clamping devices. Plastic bags usually need to be held in place with a rubber ring or wide rubber band. Make small, even pleats in the bag around the upper circumference of the ring, keeping the lower half of the appliance flange as wrinkle-free as possible. This is to prevent leakage through the folds of the plastic bag. Arrange to have the bag perpendicular to the body while the patient remains in bed. It should be placed parallel with the body when the patient is ambulatory.

14) **Attach belt** to buttons on faceplate while holding appliance steadily to skin. Pad fresh incision areas and new scars with gauze under belt. Moleskin can be affixed to the underside of the belt in region of bony prominences for additional protection and comfort. The belt should be snug, not tight. For obese patients and for patients with stomas well below the waistline, it is often necessary to wear a double belt to exert an oblique force from four points on the faceplate. Trying to "make-do" with a single belt can result in appliance displacement, more frequent changes, stoma injury, and inadequate adherence predisposing to skin excoriation from ileostomy leakage.

15) **Close end** of open-type pouch and secure.

16) **Gently rub powder** to skin under pouch and to skin-side of pouch. Place a cotton handkerchief there if patient wishes.

17) Wash permanent appliance in warm, soapy water, rinse thoroughly, and soak for five to ten minutes in a weak solution of water and vinegar, household bleach, washing soda or commercial deodorant. Hang to air dry away from sunlight and artificial heat to avoid damaging material. Do not soak appliances in strong solutions or for a long period of time as this causes deterioration.

18) **Store all ileostomy accessories** and supplies together in a dust and moisture-free place. A plastic container with a lid seal is suggested. Overnight cases and shaving kits are suitable when traveling.

Recommended References

"How to Protect Your Patients From Post-Op Skin Problems," by Michael Heindel. *RN*, January 1978:43–45.

"The Patient with an Ileostomy." *NCP Guide* #1:13, 2nd Ed, Nurseco, 1980.

Suggestions for Interviewing

Definition: An interview is a conversation with a purpose, often to obtain and/or give information.

Information Sources: The patient (client/consumer) and/or his family, friends, co-workers, teachers, employer, landlord, doctor.

General Considerations for more effective interviewing:

1) **Create a climate of comfort** (physically and psychologically):
   — See that the patient is free of pain, in a relaxed position, with a cup of liquid to drink as s/he wishes.
   — Introduce yourself with a friendly smile, tell the patient what you wish to do, and *ask his permission* to talk with him at this time.
   — Provide as much privacy as possible (draw curtain, close door or move to another room, if necessary).
   — Get on the same eye level with patient (usually by sitting down), but don't place yourself in front of a light source (sunny window or light) which will cause the patient glare and squinting.

2) **Be an attentive listener:**
   — Show interest in what the patient is saying; express respect and concern for the way s/he feels and for the effort to explain.
   — Ask broad general questions first, then narrow the subject down with more specific inquiries, such as "When did this occur?" "Can you tell me a little more about that?" or "Then, what happened?"
   — Ask open-ended questions, that is, ones which cannot be answered simply by a "yes" or "no."
   — Try to summarize or restate what the patient has said; encourage descriptions or comparisons, such as, "Was it like . . ." or "When have you felt like this before?"
   — Show acceptance (not agreement) of what s/he is saying by nodding your head or saying, "Yes . . . go on," or "Uh, hmmm . . . and?
   — Use silences to give the patient time to formulate an answer; after some wait, try re-phrasing the question or make an observation about the silence and non-verbal behavior, such as, "You seemed uncomfortable when I asked that . . ." Consider that you may have placed a barrier to further communication. Let the patient set the pace; don't press for information that s/he is unwilling or unable to divulge at this time.
   — All of the above can be considered rewards that you give the patient for giving you the information you want and need in order to help the patient. Behavior that is rewarded tends to be repeated.

3) Know and **avoid barriers to communication:**
   — Judgment is the biggest block; do not permit your values to put the patient on the defensive, "Turn him off" or make him say something that s/he really doesn't feel or believe, just to please you. Don't moralize or be philosophical.
   — Refrain from giving opinions or advice, jumping to conclusions or suggesting solutions. Don't intellectualize or try to teach patient (at this time).

— Try not to change the subject, unless it is really necessary to protect the patient or to obtain other needed information. Listen for key words, ideas, or feelings that are used more than once; then pick up on them, asking for clarification or elaboration.

— Be wary of giving false or inappropriate reassurance ("Everything will be all right") or minimizing feelings ("Everyone feels that way sometimes"). Common patient feelings are powerlessness, insecurity, loss of control, loss of dignity, and fear of pain, of the unknown, of dying, of being alone. While many patients have these feelings, it is important for the nurse to listen willingly to *this* patient's point of view and for this patient to know that you care enough to listen, without your feelings of anxiety, insecurity, etc. getting in the way.

— Keep from using stereotyped remarks and cliches, such as, "It's for your own good," or "The Doctor knows best."

4) **Plan your interview:**
— Know what kinds of information you want and how much time you have for this conversation . . . and tell your patient when you begin your interview, rather than look at your watch and tell him later.
— Use a written guide of topics, a nursing history or assessment form (see NCPG #1:46). Be sure to tell patient what you will be writing down and how the information will be used. Consider your need to know, but protect the patient's right to privacy and confidentiality.

5) **Practice** your interviewing **techniques:**
— Develop an awareness of what you are saying as well as how you are saying it. Attempt to become more sensitive to the impressions you create and the "body language" you use. Concentrate on conveying a warm, interested and caring manner.
— Analyze your own responses and negative feelings in order to better understand, accept and handle them effectively. Ask for assistance in exploring the what and why of your reactions to patients in order to get a more objective view of both the patient and yourself.
— Realize that your communications are facilitated by having open-minded, flexible and nearly accurate perceptions (judgments based on beliefs and feelings) of others.
— Remember that while *sometimes* people do not mean what they say or say what they mean, *sometimes they do;* your judgment and experiences should help you sort out the clear from the garbled messages. Keep practicing conversations, observing behavior, and validating responses to sharpen your skills. Sharpen your observation skills to notice non-verbal behavior. Be alert to posture or gestures which convey a meaning different from the words you are hearing.
— While others may be inconsistent or unexpressive of their behavior and attitudes (indeed they may even be deliberate in the inaccurate impression they wish to make), *at least* YOU may choose to facilitate open, honest communication by deliberately striving to be as expressive, consistent and truthful as you are willing to risk to be, so that growth in yourself is possible.

Recommended References
"Communication Blocks Revisited," by Sister Mary James Ramackers. *American Journal of Nursing*, June 1979:1079–1081.
"Dyadic Communication," by Mary G. Almore. *American Journal of Nursing*, June 1979:1076–1078.
"Nursing Assessment Form: RESTORING +", *NCP Guide* #1:46, 2nd Ed., Nurseco, 1980.
"Problem Patients Do Not Exisit," by Jean Scheideman. *American Journal of Nursing*, June 1979: 1082–1084.
"When Your Feelings Get In The Way," by Lynne Jungman. *American Journal of Nursing*, June 1979:1074, 1075.

Arm Exercises for the Mastectomy Patient

GOAL: The mastectomy patient's arm will be restored to full motion and usefulness; contractures, loss of function and stiffness will be prevented and muscle tone will be preserved.

General Considerations:
— Consult with doctor re: which exercises are to be taught, how often they are to be done and how long each exercise period should last. We recommend doing the beginning exercises only three times for a ten minute period twice a day; then progressing to the advanced exercises gradually, doing each exercise six times for a period of 20 minutes, three times daily.
— Teach the patient to begin with simple exercises, done slowly for short periods; then gradually add the more complex exercises, increasing the number of times performed and the length of each exercise period. Urge her to rest and breathe deeply between each exercise.
— Whenever possible, have the exercises done before a mirror so patient can be aware of correct posture and position. All exercises should begin with the patient standing up straight, shoulders back and level, abdomen flat, arms at sides, with feet six to eight inches apart for balance. Breathing should be relaxed and natural with a short pause between inhalation and exhalation.
— Use background music in a slow, rhythmic tempo to enable the patient to relax, to establish slow, swinging movements and to enjoy exercise periods.
— Explain each exercise, demonstrate it, and then assist the patient to do it correctly with your support the first few times. When possible, give her a written copy of each exercise with the number of times she is to do it in the beginning and then the amount she is to work up to after five or six weeks.

Simple Beginning Exercises:
1) Squeeze a rubber ball held in the hand, relaxing between squeezes.
2) Brush and comb the hair, keeping the neck and head as straight as possible.
3) Back scratching: with hand of unaffected side on hip for balance, swing affected arm back and with elbow bent, try to touch the shoulder blade with the finger tips.
4) Arm swinging: bending over at the waist, swing both arms forward and backward, alternately, as if swimming.
5) Arm swinging, sideward: bending over at waist, swing both arms together with hands clasped, sideward like a clock pendulum.

Advanced Exercises:

1) Rope turning: attach a length of rope to a door knob and stand about four feet away, facing door; turn rope in ever widening circles.

2) Pulley motion: place a rope (or bathrobe belt) over a shower curtain rod or tree limb; holding one end of rope in each hand, extend the arms sideways and up and down, moving the rope to slide like a pulley.

3) Raising and stretching arms: holding the ends of a golf club, yardstick or a cane, raise it above the head till arms are straight; then lower it behind the neck, raise it overhead again, then return to the waist level starting position.

4) Throw a soft, rubber or plastic ball tied to a long string, several times daily, harder and farther each day, retrieving it by drawing up the string with the fingers and hand of the affected arm.

Activities of Daily Living:

Patients are urged to progress from daily personal hygiene care to full former housework responsibilities, and then to resumption of driving or sports formerly enjoyed. Consult physician before taking on each new more strenuous activity.

Recommended References

Reach To Recovery, booklet for patients. American Cancer Society, Inc., 521 W. 57th St., New York, NY 10019.

"Teaching Patients: General Suggestions." *NCP Guide* #1:49, 2nd Ed., Nurseco, 1980.

Admitting diagnosis:

R espiration/Circulation: adequate airway? aids for breathing? cough/sputum? bleeding? edema?

E limination: bowel & bladder control & habits—any special aids?

S afety & Comfort: safety devices needed? PAIN or discomfort: physical/emotional.

T rust/Esteem/Affection: relationships with family, visitors & others. Self-image.

O rientation & Communication: state of consciousness. Language problems. Speech difficulties.

R est & Activity: sleep habits. Ambulation. Motor activities.

I nformation & Education: learning needs of patient &/or family regarding: hospital routine, procedures, treatments, self-care, etc.

N utrition: food and fluids, appetite, special diets, preferences, eating difficulties.

G eneral Observations: physical condition & appearance; signs & symptoms of illness; emotional condition and behavior.

+ the patient's perceptions of his health problems and hospitalization: Can you start at the beginning and tell me what led to his hospitalization?

RESTORING +

"an assessment tool"

NURSING DIAGNOSIS of this patient's most apparent needs/problems/concerns:

Range of Motion Exercises

GOALS: The patient will maintain joint mobility; the patient will develop muscular strength and endurance; the patient's body systems will function more efficiently; the patient's muscles will be prevented from atrophy, weakness, contracture and degeneration.

Terms:

Abduction:	Movement outward away from midline plane of body.
Adduction:	Movement toward the median plane of body.
Flexion:	Bending into a curved position.
Extension:	Stretching out into a straightened position.
Isometric Exercise:	The contraction of a muscle by tension, but without the muscle work of shortening or lengthening it.
Isotonic Exercise:	The contraction of a muscle by shortening or lengthening it through active movement.
Passive Exercise:	Muscle contraction and lengthening movements produced by another person (nurse, therapist, etc.) without the patient's effort.
Active Exercise:	Muscle movements produced by the patient's effort with little or no help from others.

General Considerations:

— Reassure the patient by telling him what you are going to do and why.

— Stress the importance of performing full range of motion exercises as soon as patient's condition permits, and on a regular, at least twice daily basis.

— Passive exercises are performed for the patient under medical orders until physician decides active exercises can be satisfactorily tolerated.

— During either passive or active exercise periods, breathing should be as normal as possible. Holding the breath is contraindicated because it can place an undue strain on the cardio-respiratory system.

— Movements are performed slowly, gently and without force. Rest is provided between each exercise, even when passively performed.

— Each exercise should be done the same number of times on both sides of the body. Do each exercise three times in the beginning and later five times.

— Perform exercises on the good side of the body, then do all the same joint movements on the affected side.

— Give the family a copy of written instructions and have them perform the exercises (with the patient) while you supervise them at least two or three times before permitting and encouraging them to do them alone.

— Massage (centripetal: toward the heart) helps circulation and reduces edema. Slow, rhythmic stroking helps relieve spasm. Heat may also be ordered to relieve pain and muscle spasm.

— Isometric exercises (i.e. alternately tightening and relaxing the muscles without moving the joints) are useful for maintaining muscle tone and increasing muscle strength which will be needed for lifting and ambulation activities. Having the patient do just 1-5 contractions per muscle group, lasting from 1-5 seconds each, with a two minute resting period in between contractions, can be most effective for strengthening purposes. Abdomen, buttocks, thighs and upper arms are the sites of choice.

Exercise List:

1) Fingers: open and close hand; spread and close fingers.
2) Thumb: bend, straighten, move in circles, touch little finger.
3) Hand: bend backward, forward, turn palm inward, outward (support wrist).
4) Elbow: bend and straighten arm.
5) Shoulder: move straight arm away from body up toward head (while supporting upper arm and hand), and then move arm back to side of body;
   — extend straight arm up into air and back to head of bed, then return to side;
   — with upper arm extended outward from body but resting on mattress, bend elbow and move lower arm forward and backward (toward head);
   — lift arm and move it across chest, then back to resting position.
6) Leg: raise and lower with knee straight (support thigh and lower leg);
   — move leg out to side, then return to body;
   — roll leg in toward other leg, then return to resting position.
7) Knee: bend leg at knee, then lower (keeping foot on bed);
   — take knee to chest, then return to straight lying position.
8) Ankle & Foot: flex foot toward leg, then extend foot ("pointing the toes");
   — turn foot outward, then inward;
   — do circles with the foot.
9) Toes: flex, extend, then spread and close toes.
10) Isometric Exercises: have the patient tense or tighten the abdominal (then buttocks, thighs and upper arms) muscles, hold for 2 or 3 seconds, then relax muscles. Rest. Repeat contractions and relaxations in other large muscle groups.

Recommended References

"Active Range-of-Motion Exercises—A Handbook," by Rudy Ciuca, Jennie Bradish and Suzanne Trombly. *Nursing 78*, August 1978:45–49.
"Passive Range-of-Motion Exercises—A Handbook," by Rudy Ciuca, Jennie Bradish and Suzanne Trombly. *Nursing 78*, July 1978:59–65.

Steps in Writing a Nursing Care Plan

Definition: A nursing care plan is the tangible end result of the nursing process, and is a hallmark of professional nursing.

General Considerations:
— **Nursing process** is the scientific method of problem-solving applied to the functions of nursing. For nurses, it is a logical method of providing patient care based on five components or steps: (1) data collection; (2) nursing diagnosis; (3) goals/objectives/expected outcomes; (4) nursing actions; and (5) evaluation of patient response.
— **Initial nursing care plans** include the first four steps; following evaluation of the patient response, **on-going plans** include all components. Each step is outlined here and is accompanied by the corresponding standard of nursing practice as defined by the American Nurses' Association (ANA).

Step 1: DATA COLLECTION

ANA Standard: "The collection of data about the health status of the client/patient is systematic and continuous. The data are accessible, communicated and recorded."

1.1 **Conduct an admission interview** with the patient and/or family/significant other(s) as soon as possible (see NCPG #1:44, "Suggestions for Interviewing.").

1.2 **Acquire additional information** from observation, physical assessment, old chart, admitting sheet, doctor, or any source possible. **Consider the kinds of information** you need in order to **START** the care plan:
- physical, emotional, and psychological states?
- patient's perception of current illness and hospitalization?
- social, cultural, economic, religious, environmental influences?
- habits and activities of daily living?
- past experiences/history of illnesses?
- what other areas will you explore?

1.3 **Write out the data** on a nursing history/interview/assessment form (See NCPG #1:46, "Restoring +" form.). Use of such a form will provide you with a tool for systematic collection of the data, as well as making it available to other personnel.

1.4 Know that **initial data collection may be limited** by one or more variables, e.g. time, patient's condition. *Do the best you can at the time;* you will have later opportunities to gather additional data.

Step 2: NURSING DIAGNOSES:

ANA Standard: "Nursing diagnoses are derived from health status data."

2.1   Nursing diagnoses are the **end products of assessment;** they are those patient needs/problems/concerns that are the *independent* functions of nursing and require nursing interventions.

2.2   Making a nursing diagnosis is the process of **interpreting** the health status data for the purpose of defining a situation. This diagnositc process has three steps (Becknell & Smith, 1975):

(1) *Extract* relevant facts and concepts from the data collected in Step 1;

(2) *Sort and clarify* this information into groups that demonstrate relationships: What pieces of data go together? Are related? Is there a logical fit between some subjective and objective data?

(3) *Interpret the data,* that is, *make a nursing diagnosis,* based on the groups or relationships you have identified.

2.3   Refer to NCPG #2:47 for the list of nursing diagnoses and the references at the end of this section.

2.4   Set **priorities** based on your nursing judgement; focus on these priority diagnoses rather than attempting to take care of all the needs/problems at once.

Step 3: GOALS/OBJECTIVES/EXPECTED OUTCOMES

ANA Standard: "The plan of nursing care includes goals derived from the nursing diagnoses."

3.1   Goals/objectives/expected outcomes (G/O/EOs) are both **long-term and short-term.**

3.2   Both are **behaviorally-stated in terms of what the patient will be doing,** not the nurse. The easiest way to do this is to use the stem, "The patient will . . ." This does not denote forcing; rather, it reflects a behaviorally-defined statement.

3.3   The **long-term G/O/EO is the desired end result of the illness or hospitalization.** Essentially, it will be a variation of *one* of the following:

(1) For the patient with an *acute* illness who has no chronicity or disability:

"The patient will return to his usual roles of (define these roles, e.g., work/family roles)."

(2) For the patient with a *chronic* illness and/or some degree of disability:

"The patient will adapt to and live within the limitations of (define the limitations and optimum level of functioning)."

(3) For the *terminally ill* patient:

"The patient will experience a peaceful and dignified death."

3.4   Each of the above long-term G/O/EOs must be **individualized to each patient**. A patient can have only one long-term G/O/EO at any given time, but it can change during hospitalization. You may not have sufficient data on admission to set a long-term G/O/EO; this may have to be done at a later date when more information is available.

3.5 **Short-term G/O/EOs are the desired end result of the nursing diagnoses.** The criteria for writing one includes that it be:

(1) *Specific:* Use specific verbs to achieve this, e.g., "The patient will *talk* . . ." "The patient will *write* . . ."

(2) *Measurable:* Include a standard of measurement, e.g., "The patient will talk about *feelings of loss of use of the arm.*" "The patient will write out a *24-hour menu for a 1500 calorie diet.*"

(3) *Realistic:* Is the G/O/EO realistic for this patient? Is it possible for the patient to achieve it?

3.6 Specify a short-term G/O/EO for **every** nursing diagnosis you have made.

Step 4: NURSING ACTIONS

ANA Standard: "The plan of nursing care includes priorities and the prescribed nursing approaches or measures to achieve the goals derived from the nursing diagnosis."

4.1 Nursing actions reflect **how** you will intervene to help the patient reach the G/O/EOs. These actions are *specific to the short-term G/O/EO* and the corresponding nursing diagnosis. As each short-term G/O/EO is being met, the results feed into achievement of the long-term one.

4.2 Prescribe your nursing actions **clearly and concisely** so that other staff using the care plan will know what you expect them to do for the patient. Instead of writing "encourage," for example, spell out what you want staff to be doing when they are "encouraging."

4.3 Determine a period of time to implement these actions before evaluation is done, e.g., "Evaluate in 3 days." Write this on the care plan card.

Step 5: EVALUATION OF PATIENT RESPONSE

ANA Standard: "The client's/patient's progress or lack of progress toward goal achievement directs reassessment, reordering of priorities, new goal setting and revision of the plan of nursing care."

5.1 **Evaluate the patient's response to the nursing actions** in relation to the short-term G/O/EO. Has the latter been achieved?

5.2 **Has the identified need/problem been resolved?** If *yes*, then direct your focus to the next priority. If progress is being made but the G/O/EO has not been reached, you may wish to continue with all actions. If there is *no* progress, then determine the cause. It could be any of the following:

(1) *The actions:* Are there other options you can try?

(2) *The short-term G/O/EO:* Is it realistic for this patient? Does it need to be changed?

(3) *The nursing diagnosis:* Is this the priority with the patient, or is there some other need/problem that is more pressing? Have new developments changed the priority?

5.3 **Revise** the care plan as necessary, according to your findings.

SUMMARY

Nursing care plans provide patients with organized, consistent care on a continuing basis. They reflect changes in the patient's health status.

Nursing process provides nurses with a professional model for providing nursing care. It is a dynamic, on-going process that reflects the independent functions of professional nursing.

Recommended References

How to Write Realistic, Workable Nursing Care Plans. A series of 4 sound filmstrips available from Nurseco, PO Box 145, Pacific Palisades, CA 90270.

"Nursing Diagnoses," *NCP Guide #2:47*, 2nd Ed., Nurseco, 1980.

Nursing Diagnosis and Intervention in Nursing Practice, by Claire Elaine Campbell. New York: John Wiley & Sons, 1978.

"Restoring +," *NCP Guide #1:46*, 2nd Ed., Nurseco, 1980.

Systems of Nursing Practice, by E. Becknell and D. Smith. Philadelphia: F.A. Davis Co., 1975.

Teaching Patients: General Suggestions

GOAL: The patient/family/significant other will develop the necessary skills, self-confident attitude and knowledge for effective control of disease and disability and for solving problems of daily living within unavoidable or recommended limitations; the patient/family/significant other will prevent, through self-care and maintenance of health, recurrence of problem or avoidable complications.

General Considerations:

— Patient education programs & departments have increased in numbers and are presently available in most hospitals, of over 150 patients, throughout the U.S.

— Nurses who believe that **patient education is** an integral part of their **nursing** role and **responsibility** can seek to fulfill their patient's teaching needs through self continuing education and by compiling a resource list of ex-patients, persons with special language skills or sign language abilities, and nursing specialists on various disease entities who will serve as consultants and helpers. Many commercial teaching aids are now available to help with patient teaching.

— Remember, **timing and patient readiness are essential to effective learning.** If patient is in a process of grief and depression over a diagnosis or impact of surgery, or is overwhelmed with fear, s/he may not hear or absorb information. S/he may even refuse to listen or to believe anything you say . . . denying a need to learn. The patient should be permitted to progress and direct own learning at own pace, even if this means that some will not be ready for self-care at discharge. Preparation of a friend or family member is suggested; transfer to a convalescent hospital may be necessary. Referral to a community health nurse is often desirable.

— Refer to NCPG #1:31, "Responses to Loss: the Grief and Mourning Process," PRN. Plan consistent care of the patient with colleagues; reinforce reality; ask questions; take time to listen.

— Consider **a written or verbal contract,** identifying what specific changes in lifestyle and behavior are needed, desired and agreed to by patient, in order to maintain the desired level of health and disease control.

— **Use** or develop an **assessment form** to guide your interview of patient and family, to assist in developing a relevant, individualized teaching plan, and to serve as a permanent record along with patient/family education record of learning attained.

— Obtain a doctor's authorization to teach patient, if this is required by hospital policy.

— Refer to NCPG #1:50, "Teaching Patients: Specific Plan for Skills and Procedures."

Nursing Actions:
  ASSESSMENT:

1) *Assess the patient/family's readiness to learn:*
   — emotional acceptance of condition, psychological adjustment, and willingness to talk about this in personal terms;
   — motivation and desire to learn, willingness and ability to modify life-style as indicated by disease/disability management or rehabilitation;
   — educational level of achievement; comprehension;
   — age and relevance of proposed teaching methods;
   — attention span; memory ability;
   — coordination (eye-hand, posture, balance, etc. as relevant);
   — vision (color and focus, acuity); hearing;
   — reading and writing ability;
   — ability to use telephone; to seek, accept and effectively use help;
   — ability to drive a car or use public transportation.

2) *Assess factors influencing teaching plan:*
   — patient's daily routine, employment conditions, family relationships, eating & sleeping patterns, travel, hobbies, use of time, responsibilities;
   — cultural and ethnic influences (dietary preferences), sexual or racial influences;
   — beliefs and attitudes re: health, illness, medical treatment;
   — is there a family member or friend who wants/needs to learn about patient's care? Can sessions be arranged to include this person, or be done at another time?
   — architectural constraints of home or living quarters, i.e. size or privacy of bathroom, number of steps, height of working surfaces, etc.

3) *Identify the important learning needs for a particular patient/family member/friend:*
   — disease pathology (cause, cure, control);
   — medication (purpose, untoward side effects, recommended dosage, administration);
   — diet (foods allowed, foods to be avoided, adaption for cultural preferences, menu selection when dining out, sample menus, food preparation);
   — activity (mental and physical rest, kind and amount of exercise, plans for leisure/recreation/sports, occupational adjustments);
   — personal health habits (smoking, drinking, coping with stress, special needs of skin, feet, hair, eyes, etc., use of assistive devices, prosthetics);
   — prevention of complications (signs and symptoms to be noted and reported, need for medical identification card);
   — community resources (address and phone number of community health agency, mutual self-help groups, vocational rehabilitation facilities, department of social services, etc.).

PLANNING:

1) Involve the family and friends (as well as the patient) in the planning, implementation and evaluation of the teaching program.
2) Establish specific, measurable, *realistic* objectives (expected outcomes); example: "Pt./S.O. can verbalize and/or demonstrate knowledge of. . . ." Arrange list of objectives in sequential steps, from simple to complex, considering also the patient's most pressing needs/problems/concerns.
3) Prepare an individualized, detailed lesson plan and assemble audio-visual teaching aids.
4) Consult sources of educational materials available for care of a given condition. Try to obtain both materials suitable for giving to patient and those recommended for teaching yourself.

IMPLEMENTATION:

1) Whenever possible, assign only one person to teach patient in order to minimize confusion, contradiction and incompleteness. Whenever possible, have that person be present when supplementary teaching is being done by a consultant specialist (dietician, volunteer ex-patient, pharmacist, etc.). Reinforce information as needed.
2) Schedule teaching sessions according to patient's receptivity (fatigue, distractibility, interest, readiness, comfort). Let patient set pace and choose topics of most interest.
3) Provide a quiet, well-ventilated, distraction-free setting for learning.
4) Provide information using visual aids; obtain feedback by asking questions; don't say, "Do you understand?" but rather, "Tell me how you can do this yourself," or, "How can you use this information in your care at home?" or, "Tell me what your situation is." This may help to reveal patient's feelings, perceptions, misconceptions and need for reiteration of facts. Correct gaps in knowledge or errors in thinking and repeat information PRN.
5) Remember that successful learning may come slowly; it takes many days of activity to regain losses of strength and endurance caused by immobility and delayed rehabilitation programs. It takes time to unlearn or relearn incorrect habits. Maintain optimism and patience. Compliment patient for effort and for each increment of learning.
6) Provide a means for patients to learn more (or reinforce what was taught). Consider supplying leaflets, written instructions, referrals to health and education service agencies, the name and number of a community health nurse or of an ex-patient successfully rehabilitated and willing to help. Attach a copy of the teaching record to the referral form.

EVALUATION:

1) Administer tests to patient to determine learning; use oral, written quizzes or return demonstrations.

2) Keep a written record of what has been **learned**, not just what was taught and by whom. Share this with nurse, family member or friend who will care for patient at home. Provide a means for the patient to evaluate his own learning and to sign record; save for use if patient is readmitted; then reactivate, update and review teaching plan.

3) Consider sending patient a letter following discharge to evaluate patient compliance and your teaching effectiveness.

Recommended References

"Forms That Facilitate Patient Teaching," by Rebecca Whitehouse. *American Journal of Nursing*, July 1979:1227–1229.

"Responses to Loss: the Grief and Mourning Process." *NCP Guide* #1:31, 2nd Ed., Nurseco, 1980.

"Teaching Patients: Specific Plan for Skills and Procedures," NCPG #1:50, 2nd Ed., Nurseco, 1980.

"What Does Your Patient Need to Know?" by Joan Kratzer. *Nursing 77*, December 1977:82–84.

Teaching Patients: Specific Plan for Skills and Procedures

Goal: The patient will be able to (state the skill or procedure) by (set a completion date).

General Considerations:
— There are many skills and procedures that patients learn from nurses, e.g. testing urine for S&A, injecting insulin, suctioning and cleaning a tracheostomy tube.
— **Optimum results** can be expected when the nurse-teacher ensures the following:
   1) inclusion of basic learning conditions;
   2) teaching the skill or procedure in specific teaching steps; and
   3) allowing for individual differences in the patient-learner.
— **Basic Learning Conditions:** the three most important for teaching skills or procedures are:
   1.1 Contiguity: The individual steps of the procedure must be taught in continuous order or sequence. You may start with the first step and work to the last one, or start with the last step and work backwards; it doesn't matter as long as the steps are **in sequence**.
   1.2   Practice: This permits the patient to rehearse the sequence until each step is learned satisfactorily. Practice will be most effective when the patient distributes it over a period of time, e.g. several times a day for several days, rather than trying to perfect the entire sequence all at once.
   1.3   Feedback: This gives the patient knowledge of how s/he is doing. It is **the most important variable** in learning, and is highly motivating to the patient. Ask the patient to give you a return demonstration of what s/he has learned; critique it and correct any errors.
— **Specific Teaching Steps:** Organizing the content to be taught in the following order facilitates presentation and comprehension:
   2.1   Emotional Acceptance of condition: If patient is denying the condition or the need to learn the skill or procedure (denial is a common behavior), read NCP Guide #1:24.
   2.2   Assessment of learning needs: What does the patient **know now**? How can you build on this? What does s/he **need to know**?
   2.3   Explanation of Terminal Behavior: Tell the patient what s/he will be able to do when the learning is completed, e.g. test urine for S&A, inject insulin, etc.
   2.4   Demonstration of Procedure: Explain and demonstrate each step **in sequence**, repeating steps PRN.
   2.5   Return Demonstration by the patient: Give encouragement and feedback; make corrections PRN.
   2.6   Verbal Restatement of each step in the procedure by the patient, in **his own** words.
   2.7   Practice by the patient until mastery of the procedure is achieved.

— **Individual Differences:** Individuals learn, accept, and cope with things at different rates. Thus, the *time* a patient requires for each step, or the entire procedure, may vary widely. Some patients will require more practice, and more explanation, than others. Be patient, and caution your patient to be likewise.

The *learning/comprehension level* will vary from patient to patient, and you will need to adjust the level of your presentation accordingly. Ensure that you use terms, words, etc. that the patient understands.

Some patients may benefit from *reading* about the procedure. If possible, supply reading materials such as booklets, pamphlets, etc.

— In **summary**, then, include the three basic learning conditions in your teaching plan, follow the specific teaching steps as outlined in (2) above, and allow for individual differences.

Recommended References
"The Patient Manifesting Denial," *NCP Guide* #1:24, 2nd Ed., Nurseco, 1980.